Heloisa Werneck de Macedo
Lusinalva L. da Silva
Patrícia F. L. Andrade

Medicinal Plants and Diabetes Mellitus

Heloisa Werneck de Macedo
Lusinalva L. da Silva
Patrícia F. L. Andrade

Medicinal Plants and Diabetes Mellitus

Treatment of Xerosis and Fissures

ScienciaScripts

Imprint

Any brand names and product names mentioned in this book are subject to trademark, brand or patent protection and are trademarks or registered trademarks of their respective holders. The use of brand names, product names, common names, trade names, product descriptions etc. even without a particular marking in this work is in no way to be construed to mean that such names may be regarded as unrestricted in respect of trademark and brand protection legislation and could thus be used by anyone.

Cover image: www.ingimage.com

This book is a translation from the original published under ISBN 978-613-9-69273-6.

Publisher:
Sciencia Scripts
is a trademark of
Dodo Books Indian Ocean Ltd. and OmniScriptum S.R.L publishing group

120 High Road, East Finchley, London, N2 9ED, United Kingdom
Str. Armeneasca 28/1, office 1, Chisinau MD-2012, Republic of Moldova, Europe
Printed at: see last page
ISBN: 978-620-8-12947-7

ACKNOWLEDGEMENTS

To God, the person most responsible for this work.

To our families, for their support, affection, patience, love and dedication, in particular to our spouses, from whom we have had every understanding and encouragement.

To our colleagues at the Fluminense Federal University, where we carried out the work that gave rise to this book, especially Professor Licínio Esmeraldo for his valuable guidance in evaluating the results of that work.

To the Diabetic Association of Nova Friburgo (ADINF), in particular to secretary Flávia Lopes for all her help and dedication, to president Mareia, to Dr Max, to all the volunteer professionals who welcomed us with so much attention and affection, and to their patients, for their pleasant interaction and teachings.

To Guilherme Rocha Macedo, for his valuable help in revising this work.

To all of you our gratitude and sincere affection.

PREFACE

Nearly 10 per cent of the world's population lives with diabetes, a disease that can lead to major complications such as chronic damage to blood vessels and nerves, mainly affecting the kidneys, retina, arteries, brain and peripheral nerves. One of the most frequent complications of diabetes is the "diabetic foot", characterised by the presence of lesions as a result of vascular and/or neurological changes peculiar to the disease. Xerosis, hyperkeratosis and fissures are complications resulting from peripheral neuronal impairment, and are risk factors for infections and ulcers, the most serious disorders affecting diabetic feet, which can lead to amputation.

Xerosis and cracks, however, are not exclusive to diabetes. Xerosis affects between 15% and 20% of the world's population and is characterised by rough, scaly skin that has lost its normal mechanical properties. The skin is unable to retain water, loses moisture faster than it gains it and can lead to the appearance of eczema, with intense itching and cracking, inflammation and secondary infection. The cracks lead to the formation of fine linear tears in the epidermis, which can crack, split and form fissures capable of reaching the dermis, causing pain and bleeding.

Treatment for xerosis is based on the repeated application of moisturisers and their use is based on solid evidence of the importance of maintaining the skin's water content. Moisturising the skin with the help of specific creams and increasing water consumption is also indicated in the treatment of cracks. Tissue repair of the skin is important for the survival of the organism, and the correct management of a skin wound and the use of appropriate medication are essential for perfect healing of the damaged area.

Empirical knowledge of the properties of plants in the treatment of various diseases, including wound healing, has accumulated over the centuries, passed down from generation to generation. Recent scientific research has revived this knowledge, seeking proof, clarification and additions that make its use safer and more effective.

In this paper we characterise the problems of xerosis and fissures, starting from the description of diabetic foot, and present the results of scientific research that today support the use of medicinal plants in their treatment.

CONTENTS

CHAPTER 1 — 5

CHAPTER 2 — 25

CHAPTER 1

DIABETES MELLITUS

1.1 The disease

Diabetes *mellitus* is a metabolic disorder of heterogeneous etiologies, characterised by hyperglycaemia and disturbances in the metabolism of carbohydrates, proteins and fats, resulting from defects in the secretion and/or action of insulin. According to the International Diabetes Federation, 8.8 per cent of the world's population aged between 20 and 79 (415 million people) live with diabetes. There are currently a growing number of people living with this disease worldwide. If current trends continue, the number of people with diabetes is projected to exceed 642 million by 2040. Around 75 per cent of cases come from developing countries, where the greatest increase is expected to occur over the coming decades. The rise in the prevalence of diabetes is associated with a number of factors, such as rapid urbanisation, a higher frequency of sedentary lifestyles, a higher frequency of being overweight, population growth and ageing, as well as the longer survival of individuals. -[14,24]

Type 1 and type 2 diabetes occur, respectively, when the body cannot produce enough of the hormone insulin or cannot utilise this insulin effectively. Type 1 is also known as insulin-dependent diabetes, childhood diabetes or immune-mediated diabetes. In this type of diabetes, the pancreas does not produce enough insulin because its cells suffer autoimmune destruction. It accounts for 5% to 10% of diabetes cases, and such patients need daily insulin injections to keep their blood glucose levels normal. Type 2 represents 90% to 95% of cases and is characterised by defects in insulin action and secretion. There is insulin resistance, leading to hyperglycaemia. This type of diabetes can occur at any age, but is usually diagnosed after the age of 40.[14,25]

Because it is not very symptomatic, diabetes *mellitus* often goes undiagnosed and untreated for many years, which favours the occurrence of its complications.[25] According to the International Diabetes Federation, 175 million people with diabetes are undiagnosed and the disease caused 5.1 million deaths in 2013. In addition, more than 79,000 children developed type 1 diabetes in the same year.[24] Quantifying the current prevalence and estimating the number of people with diabetes in the future is important because it allows us to plan and allocate resources rationally.

Data from the World Health Organisation shows that 16 million Brazilians suffer from diabetes. According to the study, the incidence rate of the disease has risen by 61.8 per cent in the last ten years. An important report is that around 50 per cent of patients are unaware of their diagnosis, and 24 per cent don't take any kind of treatment.[43,21] . More recently, it was reported that Brazil ranks 4[a] among the countries with the highest prevalence of diabetes, with 13.4 million people aged between 20 and 79 suffering from the disease.[24,21]

According to the Brazilian Society of Angiology and Vascular Surgery of Rio de Janeiro, it is estimated that every six years the number of men with diabetes *mellitus* increases by 18 per cent, and that around 20 per cent of elderly people over the age of 65 have the disease. Common major complications are chronic damage to blood vessels (vasculopathies) and nerves (neuropathies), mainly affecting the kidneys, retina, arteries, brain and peripheral nerves. They are directly related to the duration of the disease, poor glycaemic control, smoking and the presence of systemic arterial hypertension, among other factors. Diabetes *mellitus* is often not mentioned in death certificates because its complications, particularly cardiovascular and cerebrovascular complications, are the causes of death. It is estimated that 5.2 per cent of all deaths worldwide are attributed to diabetes, making it the fifth leading cause of death. A significant proportion of these deaths are premature, occurring when individuals are still contributing economically to society. According to the World Health Organisation, there is a significant increase in mortality in individuals with type 1 and type 2 diabetes *mellitus* in the presence of systemic arterial hypertension. -[14,43,53]

The direct costs of diabetes *mellitus* vary between 2.5 per cent and 15 per cent of a country's annual health budget, depending on its prevalence and the degree of complexity of the treatment available. Estimates of the direct cost for Brazil hover around 3.9 billion dollars a year. Many people with diabetes *mellitus* are unable to continue working as a result of chronic complications, or remain with some limitation in their professional performance. According to the WHO, Brazil spent R$190 billion on diabetes in 2015. This is due to limited access to good health care, with a consequent increase in the incidence of complications, disabilities and premature death.[43] One of the main causes of hospitalisation in the world for patients with diabetes *mellitus* is lower limb amputation, which is a considerable factor in incapacity, disability, early retirement and death, implying high financial costs. Diabetes is the most common cause of ulcers, infection and ischaemia. Among the most serious complications, the most frequent is non-traumatic lower limb amputation. Patients with diabetes are 15 to 30 times more likely to have an amputation than patients without diabetes.[25,50] Lack of glycaemic control, osteomyelitis, vasculopathy, peripheral neuropathy and ulcers are significant risk factors for amputations.[32]

1.2 The diabetic foot

The diabetic foot is one of the most frequent complications of diabetes *mellitus*. It is characterised by the presence of lesions as a result of vascular and/or neurological alterations peculiar to the disease, and is the most common cause of non-traumatic amputation.[32] It has multifaceted pathophysiological characteristics, resulting from the combination of chronic peripheral sensory-motor and autonomic neuropathy, associated with peripheral vascular disease, and biomechanical changes that lead to abnormal plantar pressure. Diabetic foot affects almost 6% of people with diabetes. Between 0.03% and 1.5% of patients with diabetic foot require amputation.[63,32]

The most important factors for the appearance of foot ulcers are peripheral diabetic neuropathy, misinformation about foot care, the presence of abnormal pressure points that favour calluses, deformities, peripheral vascular disease and common dermatoses (especially between the toes). Patients with a previous history of ulcers or amputations are particularly considered to be at high risk of developing new ulcers. Of all amputations in diabetic patients, 85% are preceded by a foot ulcer.[63 ,62 38]

Factors such as age, type and time of diagnosis of diabetes *mellitus,* metabolic control, smoking, alcoholism, obesity, hypertension and lack of good hygiene habits in foot care are important in terms of the risk of this complication. These factors favour ulcer formation, infection and gangrene, which can culminate in amputation.[62] .

The high human and financial cost of diabetic foot is now a worldwide concern. The control or prevention of this condition depends on widespread awareness of the need for good control of the disease and the implementation of relatively simple preventive care measures, early diagnosis and more resolute treatment in the early stages of the lesion.[9] It is essential to disseminate the concept that the diabetic foot is characterised by the presence of at least one of the following alterations: neurological, orthopaedic, vascular and infectious:[9,38]

- Sensory-motor neuropathy: gradual loss of tactile and pain sensitivity, which makes the feet vulnerable to trauma, known as "loss of protective sensation". Example: a diabetic with loss of protective sensation may no longer feel the discomfort of the repetitive pressure of a tight shoe, the pain of a sharp or cutting object on the floor or the tip of a pair of scissors when cutting their nails. It also leads to atrophy of the foot's intrinsic musculature, causing an imbalance between flexor and extensor muscles, triggering osteoarticular deformities (examples: "claw" toes, "hammer" toes, overlapping toes, prominences of the metatarsal heads, hallux valgus or bunions). These deformities alter the pressure points in the plantar region, leading to overload and skin reaction with local hyperkeratosis (callus), which, with continued walking, evolves into ulceration (plantar perforating disease). The loss of skin integrity in the situations described above is an important gateway for the development of infections, which can progress to amputation.

- Autonomic Neuropathy (Damage to the Autonomic Nervous System, in particular the Sympathetic Nerves): causes loss of vascular tone, leading to vasodilation with increased opening of arteriovenous communications and, consequently, direct passage of blood flow from the arterial to the venous network, reducing nutrition to the tissues. It also leads to anhidrosis, which causes the skin to dry out, culminating in the formation of fissures and changes in the growth and matrix of the nails, which, like chronic ulcers, are important entry points for infections.[9,36,14] ' Athlete's foot (intertrigo, chilblains) can affect the interdigital folds (between the toes) and be accompanied by onychomycosis. People with diabetes *mellitus* and a venous return deficit should take great care of their feet and avoid intertrigo, which serves as a gateway for bacterial infections in the soft tissue of the legs, causing erysipelas (skin infection).[54]

Some general precautions should be taken to prevent diabetic foot:

- *Check your feet daily;*
- *Tell your doctor if you have calluses, cracks, colour changes or ulcers;*
- *Always wear clean socks, preferably woollen or cotton;*
- *Only wear shoes that don't squeeze, preferably soft leather. Do not wear shoes without socks;*
- *New shoes should be worn little by little. Only wear them indoors for a maximum of two hours during the first few days;*
- *Never walk barefoot, even at home;*

- *Wash your feet daily with warm water and neutral soap. Avoid hot water. Dry your feet thoroughly, especially between the toes;*
- *After washing your feet, use a lanolin-based moisturiser, but don't apply it between your toes;*
- *Cut your nails straight across;*
- *Do not remove calluses or try to correct ingrown toenails. Seek professional treatment.*[38,14] .

Diabetic foot treatment involves a multidisciplinary team: endocrinologist, diabetologist, family doctor, orthopaedic surgeon, vascular and plastic surgeon, who often work together to treat and reconstruct feet and legs. Special cases may involve radiologists, pathologists and neurologists. There are treatments in hyperbaric chambers that promote oxygenation in tissues that are necrotic, resulting in very rapid regeneration and healing. Collagenase or a similar drug can be used, as well as some plant substances such as sunflower oil *(Helianthus annuus),* copaiba oil *(Copaifera langsdorffii),* barbatim *(Stryphnodendron barbatiman)* and mastic *(Schinusmolle L.).* Hydrogel dressings are a treatment option to help close diabetic foot ulcers.[15,48] Newer treatments such as growth factors applied topically to plantar ulcers, bioengineered synthetic tissues, skin grafts and mini-grafts can also be used successfully for diabetic foot ulcers as well as leg ulcers. The use of topical antibiotics and antiseptics to clean and treat foot ulcers is still a controversial topic, since infection in the diabetic foot is a life-threatening condition and must be treated incisively.[32]

1.3 Xerosis or anhidrosis

Xerosis affects between 15% and 20% of the world's population. It is a skin disorder characterised by abnormal dryness, which is common in many people and can be a symptom of certain dermatoses. It is uncomfortable, can affect the patient's quality of life and, when severe, interferes with work productivity, especially when the hands are affected. There are numerous exogenous and endogenous causes of skin xerosis: dry weather, winter, excessive exposure to water, detergents that remove lipids from the skin thus destroying the skin barrier and increasing water loss, malnutrition, marasmus, kidney failure and haemodialysis, atopy, among others. It can also occur after physiological changes that alter the blood supply to the extremities, psychological stress and contamination by microorganisms.[20] Low relative humidity and exposure to cold, dry winds lead to dehydration of the corneal layer. Factors that reduce relative humidity include space heaters and ventilating rooms with cold, dry air (winter air). This air retains little moisture when cold and becomes even drier when heated.[28,46]

The basic characteristic of xerosis is rough, scaly skin that has lost its normal mechanical properties. The stratum corneum is unable to retain water and loses moisture faster than it gains it. It is the term most often used to refer to the concept of dry skin. When severe, this condition can lead to the appearance of a type of eczema characterised by intense itching and cracking (xerotic eczema). Redness indicates inflammation and the possibility of secondary infection.[20,13,46]

Establishing a routine skin care regime is essential for keeping your skin healthy and moisturised. Unfortunately, many people underestimate the importance of this care and, as a result, dermatological problems such as xerosis appear. It is believed that the increased incidence of xerosis with advanced age is the result of changes in the keratinisation process and the lipid content of the stratum corneum, as well as the cumulative effect of environmental factors and physical damage to the stratum corneum. Also contributing are certain medications, changes in the body such as hypothyroidism, hyperthyroidism, diabetes *mellitus,* Sjogren's syndrome, and inflammatory skin conditions such as atopic dermatitis, contact dermatitis and psoriasis.[55] Xerosis, if left untreated, can lead to the development of cracks or fissures in the skin. [49,17,57,13,28,46]

Geriatric patients may have several incurable but treatable chronic diseases that affect their skin. Xerosis in older adults is multifactorial and can cause intrinsic changes in keratinisation and lipid content. Genetic predisposition, use of diuretics and similar medications and excessive use of heaters or air conditioners all contribute to this condition. Physical examination in these patients will show skin that is rough and dry to the touch, there may be peeling, and in severe cases, redness and cracks. Itching can lead to abrasions and the risk of skin infections.[60,13]

In patients with kidney problems, this alteration of the skin is common, especially in the terminal stage. It affects up to 80 per cent of dialysis patients and is an unpleasant, chronic skin manifestation with a strong negative impact on quality of life, often leading to insomnia and mood disorders.[10] In HIV patients, cutaneous manifestations are frequently observed and the prevalence of xerosis varies, reaching 73.3% to 80%.[3]

Xerosis can be caused by high blood sugar levels, and nerve damage affects the sweating process because the nerves can't receive or route the messages for sweating to occur properly.[61,14]

Diabetic patients often have skin alterations as a result of chronic hyperglycaemia. There is a 79.3 per cent prevalence of skin diseases among diabetic patients, with xerosis being the most common complication. It can affect up to 40 per cent of these patients.[20,28]

One study revealed that 82.1 per cent of diabetic patients had cracked or fissured skin and 75 per cent had xerosis, most commonly on the heels, caused by the loss of natural moisture in the stratum corneum and the skin's intercellular matrix. The sebaceous and sweat glands normally maintain skin lubrication and control the oiliness and humidity of the feet, but they become atrophied when autonomic neuropathy occurs, leading to vasodilation, which can cause xerosis with skin tears (fissures), as well as trophic changes involving nails, ligaments and joints.[47,39,22] Corneocytes are aligned parallel to each other in normal skin, but xerosis causes structural changes in these cells, resulting in a rough epidermal surface. Its presence can be an indicator of undiagnosed diabetes.[35,51] In these patients, xerosis also occurs in cases where physiological changes alter the circulatory supply to the extremities.[20]

When xerosis leads to cracks or fissures, these can serve as a gateway for infection-causing bacteria, increasing the risk of foot ulceration, which, if left unchecked, can lead to amputation. Hence the importance of examining patients' feet and offering preventive instructions and foot care, which is often forgotten.[22] They can also present pruritus and scleroderma, promoting ulceration through the development of fissures and hyperkeratosis. Their treatment is therefore paramount and must be implemented right from the start.[42,20,51,22] The basis of treatment is rehydration and skin repair, which are very important for recovering the epidermal barrier function.[42,13]

Infection is a limb-threatening condition and is considered an immediate cause of amputation in 25 to 50 per cent of diabetic patients. Retrospective clinical studies of these patients with foot infections show progression to minor amputations in 24 to 60 per cent of cases and to major amputations in 10 to 40 per cent of cases. A prospective study on deep infection reported an amputation rate of 52 per cent.[12]

Approximately 50% of all reasons for hospitalisation among diabetics are foot-related problems. Xerosis, hyperkeratosis and fissures are complications resulting from peripheral neuronal impairment. However, these complications are risk factors for infections and ulcers, the most serious disorders affecting diabetic feet, which can lead to amputation.[28]

In order to avoid the formation of cracks in the skin of diabetics, in addition to treating dry skin, it is necessary to have good eating habits, control blood glucose, take care of personal hygiene and especially take care of the feet, wearing appropriate shoes, constantly observing them and reporting any abnormalities to the doctor, as it is in this area that cracks appear.

Patients can minimise the effect of xerosis by increasing the humidity of the environment, modifying bath products and using emollients to replace the lipid components of the skin. Care must be taken to avoid sensitising the skin with substances that cause hypersensitivity, such as lanolin and parabens, which are commonly found in some products. Otherwise, cracks can form, which are often painful and can act as a gateway for microorganisms. Acne, eczema, dermatitis, warts and fungal infections were considered the most common skin problems in Americans and Arabs, but xerosis was considered one of the most persistent and serious problems.[16,20,46]

The treatment for xerosis is the repeated application of moisturisers and their use is based on solid evidence about the importance of maintaining the skin's water content. Although the skin on the plantar surface is very thick, highly visco-elastic, used to high levels of tension, compression and the impact applied to it, problems arise when the skin becomes dry and loses its elastic property.[5,8]

Effectively moisturising the skin of the feet is an important strategy for preventing ulcers and maintaining foot health. Moisturisers and emollients are effective in improving these disorders and restoring the barrier function of the epidermis, and are therefore indicated for the treatment of xerosis through constant use.[20,41,28]

Topical products such as emollients and moisturisers are effective in repairing the epidermal barrier function and improving xerosis. Few studies have been carried out on diabetic patients evaluating treatments that can help correct alterations in the functional and mechanical properties of their skin.[20]

Patients should be instructed to avoid creams and lotions that contain alcohol, perfumes or colourants, as these can increase dryness and lead to greater skin irritation. In addition, any skin changes can increase sensitivity to the sun and therefore patients should be advised to use sunscreen with a protection factor of 15 or more and avoid exposure to the sun when possible.[17]

Most cases of xerosis respond to treatment with moisturisers, but if the dryness of the skin is particularly severe or seems to worsen after at least seven days of self-treatment, patients should seek medical attention.[55] Studies have shown that there are creams based on urea, carnosine and arginine for the treatment of these lesions, moisturising the skin.[19,20] However, studies on herbal medicines developed for this purpose, mainly using essential oils as the active ingredient, are quite scarce in the literature.

Emollients such as glycerine and propylene glycol are commonly used to treat xerosis in diabetic patients, in combinations with water, oils and fats, to help moisturise the skin and restore oil lost due to dryness. When used correctly, they are an essential part of dermatitis control and help the skin heal.[51,8] A study on patients with diabetes and xerosis using a formula containing oil, water, ceramide and glyceryl also showed good results in moisturising the skin and eliminating xerosis.[59,28]

The application of formulations containing oils and hygroscopic elements helps to restore the barrier, allowing adequate water levels to be maintained. The effect is felt immediately after application, with an improvement in common signs of xerosis, such as roughness and flaking.[1,28] Canola oil (*Brassica napus L. Var.*) is considered an important emollient for the skin[26] as well as *Aloe vera,* to moisturise skin with xerosis and also to replace the lipid components lost by the skin.[30]

Daily moisturisation is a vital part of the treatment of patients with atopic dermatitis and xerosis. The choice of moisturising cream and its composition determine whether the treatment strengthens or deteriorates the skin's barrier function, which can have consequences for the outcome of the treatment of xerosis and dermatitis. Despite the relief of visible symptoms of skin dryness, abnormal high transepidermal water loss has been reported even with the use of certain moisturisers, while others improve the skin's barrier function. That's why it's important to choose the right product for treatment, and to do so you need to know its composition.

1.4 Skin cracks or fissures and wound healing

Fissures determine the formation of fine linear tears in the epidermis, which can crack, split and form fissures capable of reaching the dermis, causing pain and bleeding, also known as cracks, ragdia, fissures or cracks. They can be defined as small cracks or fissures in the calloused skin of the hands or feet, caused by linear loss of the epidermis and dermis, mainly in areas of skin folds or creases. They are elementary lesions and form part of the "tissue loss" group. Fissures can vary in thickness, some lesions affect the skin only superficially and others can even reach deep tissue.[58,22]

These lesions are the result of the elimination or destruction of skin tissues, basically caused by the loss of skin elasticity. Determining factors for the appearance of cracks in the skin are: skin dryness, age (naturally responsible for the appearance and increase in the number of folds in the skin), eating habits (for example, uric acid, when not eliminated by the body, attacks the joints of the hands and feet, causing lesions), amount of water ingested (a minimum of 5% in litres is recommended, of body weight), the use of medication (this can directly affect the elasticity of the skin), exposure of the skin to chemical aggressions and the soil (this intensifies the dryness of the skin, damages and contaminates wounds), the use of unsuitable socks and shoes and obesity.[40,22]

The main causes of cracks are climate change: in dry and cold environments the skin loses water and thus becomes more dehydrated. Dehydration causes dry skin to flake off and become brittle, as it is essential for the skin's water balance and for maintaining healthy skin. Water depletion can lead to complications such as cracks and sores. Another cause of cracks is chemical aggression. The use of soaps and detergents removes fat from the skin, affecting the lipid mantle that helps maintain the skin's natural moisture, leaving it unprotected. Diabetes *mellitus* can also be a cause of cracks since high blood glucose levels over a long period can damage blood vessels and prevent blood from reaching the area. This reduction in circulation can weaken the skin and contribute to the appearance of wounds and make healing more difficult. Obesity is also a factor in the development of cracks because, due to excess weight, the skin thickens in a defence reaction to better withstand pressure. Being just 5kg overweight already puts a strain on the feet.[40,11] The xerosis and fissures that affect people with diabetes can lead to the formation of ulcers and the loss of lower limbs due to lack of treatment.[6,22,29,11]

In the treatment of cracks, it is recommended to increase water consumption and moisturise the feet with the help of specific creams such as urea cream, which is an important humectant, especially when the skin is extremely dry, but in concentrations above 20% it can become keratolytic and dehydrating.[6] As the body's first protective barrier against external agents, the skin is subject to constant aggression. Its tissue repair is therefore important for the body's survival. However, the correct management of a skin wound and the use of appropriate medication are essential for perfect healing of the injured area.[52,11,4,23]

The healing process is a complex process that basically takes place in three phases, as follows:

- Inflammatory phase: the initial events of the repair process are initially aimed at plugging the vessels. The first response is vasoconstriction. This is followed by the formation of a platelet-rich thrombus, which temporarily plugs the endothelial lesion. This thrombus is infiltrated by fibrin, turning into a fibrinous thrombus, where erythrocytes are captured, forming the red thrombus. The mediators released by activated platelets guide the migration of inflammatory cells (polymorphonuclear cells, macrophages and lymphocytes) to the site of the injury;

- Fibroblastic and extracellular matrix deposition phase: there is an increase in the number of activated fibroblasts at the site and collagen is produced. The extracellular matrix begins to be replaced by stronger and more elastic connective tissue (fibroplasia). This process is accompanied by angiogenesis, which initiates the formation of granulation tissue;

• Remodelling phase: the granulation tissue is enriched with more collagen fibres and begins to take on the appearance of a fibrotic mass characteristic of a scar, and the extracellular matrix slowly matures and remodels.[44,23,29,11 ,34]

In people with diabetes, these phases can be altered and other interventions are needed to help the healing process, which can be compromised due to infectious processes in the lesion or metabolic alterations related to diabetes. [2,18,11,48]

Hyperglycaemia causes damage to various tissues in the body. Most of the complications are related to problems in the blood vessels which, as well as containing glucose, carry nutrients and collect toxins from the body's tissues. These vessels can be blocked or damaged by excess glucose, which causes damage to the organs they irrigate and impairs the repair and healing process. This process in these patients is slower and more precarious due to vascular damage, reduced collagen synthesis and damage to connective tissue. Diabetes *mellitus* leads to extensive skin damage. Healing is often not complete and causes chronic wounds, which can lead to irreversible damage.[311148] The difficulty in healing may be due to compromised blood perfusion, preventing an adequate supply of oxygen, nutrients and antibiotics, especially to the lower limbs. This leads to disorganisation of the initial stages of repair, delaying the process of tissue regeneration.[2,34]

People with diabetes *mellitus* are vulnerable to a series of complications of a metabolic nature and/or of an infectious, viral and fungal origin. The feet are the biggest targets of the chronic complications to which diabetics are subject. They are very susceptible to serious damage and are difficult to heal.

Injuries occur through an association of ulcerations, infections and gangrene, with long healing processes.[33,37,27]

Chronic wounds are a serious public health problem, affecting around 1% of the world's population, regardless of gender, age or race. Despite a multidisciplinary approach, the management of patients with chronic wounds is a major challenge. In addition to its profound effect on the quality of life of affected individuals, around 2% of the health budget is allocated to wound care.[84]

Wound treatment seeks rapid closure of the lesion in order to achieve a functional and aesthetically satisfactory scar. The cost of treating pathologies related to scar deficiency increases the importance of research into drugs capable of interacting with damaged tissue in order to speed up the process. This is important, for example, in the case of diabetic foot ulcers where healing is delayed. -[31,56,11,28,4]

There are several studies that prove the effectiveness of using products that help repair and heal skin lesions, such as the use of trans-retinoic acid in tissue repair and the production of type I pro-collagen. This retinoid offers excellent results on severely damaged skin, but causes great irritation to the skin of most individuals. These irritations can counteract its beneficial effects, causing an increase in the inflammatory process, making the individual more prone to wounds and leading to treatment abandonment.[7]

Urea is an organic compound that has been used clinically to treat dermatological diseases for over a century. Urea is a powerful emollient and keratolytic agent, making it effective for treating conditions associated with xerosis and scaly skin, as it is a widely used moisturiser due to its ability to retain water in the epidermal barrier (hygroscopy). Its natural presence in the stratum corneum is evidenced in the literature, making up around 7% of the natural moisturising factor. Studies have reported that the 10 per cent concentration is significantly better than other concentrations, which can cause adverse symptoms such as burning and tingling.[45,1]

1.5 Bibliography

1. ADDOR, F. A. S.; SCHALKA, S.; PEREIRA, V. M. C. et al. Correlation between the moisturising effect of urea at different application concentrations: clinical and corneometric study. Surgical Cosmetic, 1(1): 5-9, 2009.

2. ANDRADE, M. G. L.; CAMELO, C. N.; CARNEIRO, J. A. et al. Evidence of changes in the burn healing process in diabetic individuals: a literature review. Rev Bras Queimaduras, 12(1): 42-48, 2013.

3. ATADOKPEDE, F. H.; ADEGBIDI, J. J.; SEHONOU, C. et al. Prevalence of xerosis, eczema and a hair and nail abnormalities in plwha in cotonou, Benin. Int J Dermatol, 1: 48-50, 53-55, 2012.

4. ATAIDE A. J.; CEFALI L. C.; CROISFELT F. M. et al. Natural actives for wound healing: A review. Phytother Res, 2018.

5. BAALHAM, P.; BIRCH, I.; YOUNG, M. *et al.* Xerosis of the feet: a comparative study on the effectiveness of two moisturisers. Br J Community Nurs, 16(12): 591-592, 594-597, 2011.

6. BEGA, Armando. Treatise on podiatry. 2. ed. São Paulo: Yendis, 2013. 416 p.

7. BHAGAVATHULA, N.; WAGNER, R. L.; SILVA, M. *et al.* A combination of curcumin and ginger extract improves abrasion wound healing in corticosteroid-damaged hairless skin. Wound rep reg, 17(3): 360-366, 2009.

8. BORALEVI F.; MELEDIE N'DJONG AP.; YAO YOBOUE P. et al. Regression of cutaneous xerosis with emollient treatment in sub-Saharan African patients. Int J Dermatol, 56(4):467-473, 2017.

9. CAIAFA, J. S.; CASTRO, A. A.; FIDELIS, C. *et al.* Comprehensive care for diabetic foot patients. J Vasc Bras, 10(4): 1-31,2011.

10. CASTELLO, M.; MILANI, M. Efficacy of topical hydrating and emollient lotion containing 10% urea isdin® plus dexpanthenol (ureadin rx 10) in the treatment of skin xerosis and pruritus in haemodialyzed patients: an open prospective pilot trial. G ital dermatol venereol, 146(5): 321-325, 2011.

11. CHENG K. Y .; LIN Z. H .; CHENG Y. P. *et al.* Wound Healing in Streptozotocin-Induced Diabetic Rats Using Atmospheric-Pressure Argon Plasma Jet. Sei Rep, 8: 12214, 2018.

12. INTERNATIONAL CONSENSUS ON DIABETIC FOOT. Available at: http://dms.ufpel.edu.br/ares/handle/123456789/182. Accessed on: 13 Aug. 2018.

13. CRUZ R. A. O.; ACIOLY C. M. C.; ARAÚJO A. A. et al. Cutaneous xerosis

in the elderly: the importance of specialised nursing care. UNINGÁ, 49(1): 107-112, 2016.

14. GUIDELINES OF THE BRAZILIAN DIABETES SOCIETY, 2018. Available at : https://www.diabetes.org.br/profissionais/images/2017/diretrizes/diretrizes-sbd-2017-2018.pdf. Accessed on: 20 Aug. 2018.

15. DUMVILLE, J. C.; 0'MEARA, S.; DESHPANDE, S. et al. Hydrogel dressings for healing diabetic foot ulcers. Cochrane Database Syst Rev, 7(9): 1-54, 2013.

16. EL-ESSAWI, D.; MUSIAL, J. L.; HAMMAD, A. et al. A survey of skin disease and skin-related issues in Arab Americans. J Am Acad Dermatol, 56(6): 933-938, 2007.

17. ESPER, P.; GALE, D.; MUEHLBAUER, P. What kind of rash is it?: deciphering the dermatologic toxicities of biologic and targeted therapies. Clin J Oncol Nurs, 11(5): 659-666, 2007.

18. FAN B.; WANG T.; BIAN L. *et al.* Topical Application of Tat-Rac1 Promotes Cutaneous Wound Healing in Normal and Diabetic Mice. Int J Biol Sei, 14(10):1163-1174, 2018.

19. FEDERICI, A.; FEDERICI, G.; MILANI, M. An urea and carnosine based cream (Ureadin Rx Db ISDIN) shows greater efficacy in the treatment of severe xerosis of the feet in type 2 diabetic patients in comparison with glycerol-based emollient cream. BMC Dermatol, 12(1): 16, 2012.

20. FEDERICI, A.; FEDERICI, G.; MILANI, M. Use of a urea, arginine and carnosine cream versus a Standard emollient glycerol cream for treatment of severe xerosis of the feet in patients with type 2 diabetes: a randomised, 8 month, assessor-blinded, controlled trial. Curr Med Res Opin, 31(6): 1063-9, 2015.

21. FIOCRUZ, 2018. Diabetes incidence rate grew 61.8% in the last 10 years. Available at: https://portal.fiocruz.br/noticia/taxa-de- incidence-of-diabetes-grew-618-in-the-last-10-years. Accessed on: 20 Aug. 2018.

22. GIN H.; RORIVE M.; GAUTIER S. et al. Treatment by a moisturiser of xerosis and cracks of the feet in men and women with diabetes: a randomized, double-blind, placebo-controlled study. Diabet Med, 34(9): 1309-1317, 2017.

23. HOSSEINKHANI A.; FALAHATZADEH M.; RAOOFI E. *et al.* An Evidence-Based Review on Wound Healing Herbal Remedies From Reports of Traditional Persian Medicine. J Evid Based Complementary Altern Med, 2017.

24. INTERNATIONAL DIABETES FEDERATION (IDF). IDF Diabetes Atlas, 6th edn, 2018. Available at: http://www.idf.org/diabetesatlas. Accessed on: 18 Aug. 2018.

25. LIMA C. L. J.; FERREIRA T. M.; OLIVEIRA P. S. *et al.* Characterisation of users at risk of developing diabetes: a cross-sectional study. Rev Bras Enferm [Internet], 71(1): 516-523, 2018.

26. LODÉN, M. Effect of moisturisers on epidermal barrier function. Clin Dermatol, 30(3): 286-296, 2012.

27. MAHBOUBI M.; TAGHIZADEH M .; KHAMECHIAN T. et al. The Wound Healing Effects of Herbal Cream Containing *Oliveria Decumbens* and *PelargoniumGraveolens* Essential Oils in Diabetic Foot Ulcer Model. World. J Plast Surg, 7(1): 45-50, 2018.

28. MARTINI J.; HUERTAS C.; TURLIER V. et al. Efficacy ofan emollient cream in the treatment of xerosis in diabetic foot: a double-blind, randomised, vehicle-controlled clinical trial. J Eur Acad Dermatol Venereol, 31(4):743-747, 2017.

29. MARTINO O.; TITO A.; DE LUCIA A. et al. Hibiscus syriacus Extract from an Established Cell Culture Stimulates Skin Wound Healing. Biomed Res Int, 2017.

30. MENDONÇA, F. A. S.; PASSARINI, JÚNIOR, J. R.; ESQUISATTO, M. A. *et al.* Effects of the application of Aloe vera (L.) and microcurrent on the healing of wounds surgically induced in Wistar rats. Acta Cir Bras, 24(2): 150-155, 2009.

31. MENDONÇA, R. J.; NETTO, J. C. Cellular Aspects of Scarring. An Bras Dermatol, 84(3): 257-262, 2009.

32. MISHRA, S. C.; CHHATBAR K. C; KASHIKAR A.; MEHNDIRATTA A. Diabetic foot. BMJ, 359, 2017.

33. MONTES, L. V.; BROSEGHINI, L. P.; ANDREATTA, F. S. *et al.* Evidence for the use of copaiba oil-resin in wound healing - a systematic review. Nature, 7(2): 61-67, 2009.

34. MORESKI D. B.; BUENO F. G.; LEITE-MELLO E. V. S. Healing action of medicinal plants: a review study. Arq. Ciênc. Saúde UNIPAR, 22(1): 63-69, 2018.

35. MORGAN, N. What you need to know about xerosis in patients with diabetic feet. Wound Care, 2(4), 2013.

36. NASCIMENTO O. J. M.; PUPE C. C. B.; CAVALCANTI E. B. U. Diabetic neuropathy. Rev Dor. São Paulo, 17(1): 46-51, 2016.

37. NAYAK, B. S.; RAJU, S. S.; RAO, A. V. Wound healing activity of Matricaria recutita L. extract. J Wound Care, 16(7): 298-302, 2007.

38. NETO G. R. A.; TEIXEIRA T. F. S.; ROCHA F. C. et al. Diabetic foot assessment in primary care: an integrative review. REAS, 12: 166- 1170, 2018.

39. NOGUEIRA, M. Hydrosis. RevistaPodologia, (14): 11,2007.

40. NUNES, J. C.; MARCELINO, J.; NOVOTNY, V. R. The main causes of foot cracks, 2011. Available at: http://SiaibibO1.univali.br/pdf/ Jessica Nunes, Jessica Marcelino.pdf. Accessed on: 21 July 2013.

41. O'SULLIVAN, G.; FOTINOS, C.; ST. ANNA, L. ET AL. ANNA, L. et al. What treatments relieve painful heel cracks? JFP, 61(10): 622, 2012.

42. ONSELEN, J. V. Dry skin condition an evidenced-based focus on natural oatmeal emollients. JMPHC, 21(2): 31-37, 2011.

43. WORLD HEALTH ORGANISATION (OMS), 2018. Available at: https://www.paho.org/bra/index.php?option=com_content&view=article&id=394:diabetes-mellitus&Itemid=463. Accessed on: 18 Aug. 2018.

44. ORYAN A.; MOHAMMADALIPOUR A.; MOSHIRI A. *et al.* Topical Application of Aloe vera Accelerated Wound Healing, Modelling, and Remodeling: An Experimental Study. Ann Plast Surg± 77(1): 37-46, 2016.

45. PAN, M.; HEINECKE, G.; BERNARDO, S. *et al.* Urea: a comprehensive reviewof the clinical literature. Dermatol Online J, 19(11): 1-16, 2013.

46. PARKER J.; SCHARFBILLIG R.; JONES S. Moisturisers for the treatment of foot xerosis: a systematic review. J Foot Ankle Res, 10: 9, 2017.

47. PAVIC, T.; KORTING, H. C. Xerosis and callus formation as a key to the diabetic foot syndrome: Dermatologic view of the problem and its management. J Dtsch Dermatol Ges, 4: 935-941, 2006.

48. PÉREZ-RECALDE M.; RUIZ ARIAS I. E.; HERMIDA É. B. Could essential oils enhance biopolymers performance for wound healing? A systematic review. Phytomedicine, 38:57-65, 2018.

49. PROKSCH, E.; LACHAPELLE, J. M. The management of dry skin with topical emollients--recent perspectives. J Dtsch Dermatol Ges, 3(10): 768-774, 2005.

50. SADRIWALA A. D.; GEDAM B. S.; AKHTAR M. A. Risk factors of amputation in diabeticfoot infections. Int Surg J, 5(4): 1399-1402, 2018.

51. SEITE, S.; KHEMIS. A.; ROUGIER, A. *et al.* Importance of treatment of skin xerosis in diabetes. J Eur Acad Dermatol Venereol, 25(2): 607-609, 2011.

52. SHIMIZU, B. J.; EURIDES, D.; BELETTI, M. E. *et al.* 5% barbatim extract in hydroxyethylcellulose gel applied to experimentally produced skin wounds in mice. Vet Not, 15(1): 21-27, 2009.

53. BRAZILIAN SOCIETY OF ANGIOLOGY AND VASCULAR SURGERY OF RIO DE JANEIRO (SBACVRJ). The number of men with diabetes is growing. Available at: http://www.sbacvrj.com.br/paciente/br/ler/612/85/Not%C3%ADcias/cresce-numero-de-homens-com-diabetes. Accessed on: 18 September 2013.

54. BRAZILIAN SOCIETY OF DERMATOLOGY, 2017. Available at:

http://www.sbdrs.org.br/diabeticos-precisam-ter-atencao-redobrada-com-a-pele. Accessed on: 20 Aug. 2018.

55. TERRIE, Y.; C. Itchy, Scratchy Skin: Preventing and Managing Xerosis. BSPharm, 79(6): 18-19, 2013.

56. THAKUR, R.; JAIN, N.; PATHAK, R. *et al.* Practices in Wound Healing Studies of Plants. Evid Based Complement Alternat Med, 2011(2011): 1-17, 2011.

57. *VAEGELI,* D. The role of emollients in the care of patients with dry skin. Nurs Stand, 22(7): 62-68, 2007.

58. VIANA, Maria Auxiliadora Fontenelle. Podological atlas. Minas Gerais: FAPI, 2011.

59. WEBER, T. M.; KAUSCH, M.; RIPPKE, F. et al. Treatment of xerosis with a tropical formulation containing glyceryl glucoside, natural moisturising factors, and ceramide. J Clin Aesthet dermatol, 5(8): 29-39, 2012.

60. WHITE-CHU, E. F.; REDDY, M. Dry skin in the elderly: complexities of a common problem. Clin Dermatol, 29(1): 37-42, 2011.

61. WOOLLEY, E. Diabetes and Skin Problems. Medical Review Board, 2012.

62. YILDIZ A. P.; ÕZDIL T. O.; DIZBAY M. et al. Peripheral arterial disease increases the risk of multidrug-resistant bacteria and amputation in diabetic foot infections. Turk J Med Sei, 48(4): 845-850, 2018.

63. ZHANG P1, LU J1, JING Y. et al. Global epidemiology of diabetic foot ulceration: a systematic review and meta-analysis. Ann Med, 49(2): 106-116, 2017.

CHAPTER 2

MEDICINAL PLANTS IN THE TREATMENT OF DERMATOLOGICAL DISEASES

2.1 Current knowledge

The products used for skin repair must have peculiar structural and functional requirements: they must have no antigenotoxicity; they must not provoke an inflammatory reaction; they must facilitate colonisation of the stromal cells and the synthesis of glycoproteins; they must encourage the migration and differentiation of epithelial cells. These properties can be translated as efficacy, safety and versatility, which together also provide patient comfort, ease of application or removal, medical safety and a positive cost/benefit ratio with the clinical use of the product. [68,75,35]

For centuries, medicinal plants have been used as alternatives for the treatment of various dermatological diseases, especially those with scarring processes that are difficult to resolve. The World Health Organisation defines a medicinal plant as any plant that contains, in one or more organs, substances that can be used for therapeutic purposes or that are precursors to semi-synthetic drugs. The difference between a medicinal plant and a herbal medicine lies in the preparation of the plant for a specific formulation, which characterises a herbal medicine. According to the Health Surveillance Secretariat, in its ordinance no. 6 of 31 January 1995, a herbal medicine is any medicine that is technically obtained and prepared using exclusively plant raw materials for prophylactic, curative or diagnostic purposes, with benefits for the user.

Over the centuries, products of plant origin have formed the basis for the treatment of various diseases, due to the knowledge of a particular plant's properties being passed down from generation to generation.

Its use in the wound healing process has been mentioned since prehistoric times, when plants and plant extracts were used in the form of poultices to stop bleeding and promote healing, and many of these plants were ingested to act systemically. It can therefore be said that medicine, as we know it today, was only made possible by the recovery of healing methods and empirical knowledge used thousands of years ago.[81,47,59,11]

In ancient Egypt, inflammatory processes were treated with an extract obtained from the bark of the willow tree *(Salix alba, Salix alba Caerulea, Salix sepulcralis Chrysocoma, Salix Tristis, Salix babylonica, Salix matsudana)*, which was used to treat suppurating wounds and later proved to have anti-inflammatory properties.[81,8]

Nowadays, even in developed countries, people are looking for alternative therapies for wound healing instead of modern antibiotic and corticoid therapies.[47,59] This is due to the side effects that the use of these drugs can have.[50,70]

Due to the lower occurrence of these unwanted effects compared to synthetic drugs, approximately 60% of the world's population uses plants almost exclusively for medication, and natural products have been recognised as an important source of therapeutically effective medicines.[45]

Among the bioactive substances that can be found in the various parts of a plant are alkaloids, saponins, tannins, glycosides, flavonoids and essential oils. They are therefore an unlimited source of potentially active substances and many of them are used to help promote healing and angiogenesis. They are considered raw materials for the development of new molecules and drugs. Although popular knowledge has contributed significantly to understanding the effects of medicinal plants, the active principles, mechanism of action and toxicity of many of them are still poorly understood, justifying scientific research to prove their efficacy. [34,59,83]

Plants have various chemical constituents with antimicrobial and healing potential. They are alternatives for treating infected wounds. However, popular use is not enough to validate them as effective and safe.[61]

Although the pharmaceutical industry has made considerable advances in the availability of drugs capable of stimulating the healing process, only 1 to 3 per cent of all the drugs listed in Western pharmacopoeias are intended for use on the skin or wounds. Of these, at least 1/3 are obtained from medicinal plants. In recent years, research into natural products as aids in the healing process has intensified.[28]

Many herbal moisturisers have been studied and proven to be effective in helping to regenerate the skin, muscles and lymphatic function, and are particularly useful for treating ageing skin.[71] There are also reports on the use of medicinal plants used to make creams, gels and oils, which act to help heal and heal wounds.[36,85 ,48]

Some healing herbs improve blood clotting, fight infection and speed up healing. They have been used to prepare products for this purpose.[98,11,83] Several of them have represented a new attempt at wound healing, for example in the case of diabetic foot ulcers. The use of a natural cream made up of a mixture of various herbs *(Aloe vera lank, Pandanus odaratissimus, Curcuma longa, Cocos nucifera, Glycyrrhiza glabra, Musa paradisíaca)* was compared with silver sulphadiazine cream, a bactericide derived from sulphamides, in the treatment and healing of wounds.

on the skin of type 2 diabetic patients. The product developed generated good results in the reduction of the patients' wounds, collagen synthesis, as well as microbicidal and anti-inflammatory action.[71 ,69,8,47,59].

Different plants have been used successfully to repair tissue and heal wounds. *Aloe vera* (L.) Burm. f. (aloe), *Coronopu didymus* (mastruz), *Arnica Montana* L. (arnica), *Orbignya phalerata* (babassu), *Stryphnodendron adstringens* Martius (barbatimão), *Caesalpinia ferrea* Martius (Qucá), *Chenopodium ambrosioides* L. (Santa Maria grass), *Triticum vulgana* (wheat),

Tabernaemontana catharharensens (wheat). (Santa Maria grass), *Triticum vulgare* (wheat), *Tabernaemontana catharinensis* (jasmine), *Calendula officinalis* (marigold), *Helianthus annus* (sunflower), *Catharanthus roseus* L. (vinca rosea), *Schinus terebinthifolius* Raddi (mastic) and *Tabebuia avellanedae* (purple ipe) are plants that have been successfully used for this purpose.[59]

Jatropha curcas, Aloe barbadensis and *Centella asiatica* exhibit antimicrobial, antioxidant, antifungal and anti-inflammatory properties.[45,11] .

Olive oil (*Olea europaea),* oregano *(Origanum vulgare)* and sage *(Salvia officinalis L.)* are species that have been used to treat inflammatory diseases and heal skin wounds in traditional Turkish medicine. In India, the plants most commonly used for these purposes are *Aloe vera, Azadirachta indica, Carica papaya, Centella asiatica, Celosia argentea, Cinnamomum zeylanicum, Nelumbo nucifera, Ocimum sanctum, Phyllanthus emblica, Plumbago zeylanica, Pterocarpus santalinus, Terminalia arjuna* and *Terminalia chebula.*[94,47,8] '.

Delayed wound healing can be a consequence of diabetes *mellitus,* immunological diseases, ischaemia and venous stasis. Studies with an aqueous extract of the leaf of *Hippophae rhamnoides* L. showed an improvement in the healing of skin wounds in rats. The properties of *Aloe vera* L. and *Curcuma longa* L. in the healing process have also been demonstrated and studied experimentally in various animal models. A formulation made with a combination of the aqueous extracts of freeze-dried leaves of *Hippophae rhamnoides* L., *Aloe vera* L. and the ethanolic extract of the rhizome of *Curcuma longa* L. was tested in order to assess its effectiveness in healing diabetic and chronic wounds in rats. The result was complete wound healing, which was much better in diabetic wounds compared to chronic wounds.[44,20,11]

A study showed the effectiveness of a herbal cream containing essential oils of *Pelargonium graveolens* and *Oliveria decombens* separately and together in diabetic rats with ulcers. As a result, it reported that there was a significant reduction in the size of the wounds when the oils were applied separately, but together the oils provided greater tissue repair.[53]

Morinda citrifolia Linn (Indian mulberry) is a small evergreen tree that traditional Polynesian healers use for many purposes, including healing skin wounds. An ethanolic extract of its leaves was prepared to evaluate its wound healing activity in rats, using wound excision models. The animals that used the extract showed a 71 per cent reduction in wound area, while the controls that used water showed a 57 per cent reduction. *Morinda tinctoria* Roxb is an effective healing agent for treating internal and external wounds.[65,83]

Hibiscus rosa sinensis Linn. (Malvaceae) is a shrub widely cultivated as an ornamental plant. The leaves and flowers are known to help heal ulcers. The healing activity of this plant was observed and proven in a study carried out on Wistar albino rats, using wound excision and incision models. The results showed that the extract increased cell proliferation and collagen synthesis at the wound site. The wounds treated with the extract healed much faster and had a better rate of epithelialisation and wound contraction. *Hibiscus syriacus* stimulates the expression of biomarkers relevant to skin regeneration and moisturisation, counteracting the molecular pathways that lead to skin damage and ageing.[18,56]

Matricaria recutita L., *Matricaria chamomilla, Chamomilla chamomile* and *Matricaria suaveolens,* popularly called chamomile, have been used for centuries as medicinal plants, mainly for injuries and skin problems. In Germany, for example, chamomile is used to treat wounds and its effectiveness has been reported and confirmed in several studies. The flower extract has pro-inflammatory, healing and platelet aggregation enhancing activity when applied topically. [65,6,10,54]

Rafflesia hasseltii is a plant found in Malaysia that has skin healing properties, promotes angiogenesis and collagen synthesis. However, this plant is very rare and therefore little used.[1,101]

A study carried out at the University of Michigan Medical School obtained good results with the use of a product made with glycerol extract enriched with ginger root *(Zingiber officinalis) and* turmeric *(Curcuma longa),* compared to retinoids. Unlike these, the extract did not promote skin irritation. Ginger, in particular, demonstrated angiogenesis-promoting properties, improving wound healing. It also showed antioxidant and anti-inflammatory properties. Turmeric showed antioxidant properties, promoted collagen synthesis, reduced levels of matrix metalloproteinases and promoted skin healing.[17,31]

Studies have tested the antimicrobial, antioxidant and healing activity of *Pongamia Pinnata* leaf extract. As a result, the authors reported that this extract exhibited significant antimicrobial activity against *Staphylococcus aureus, Staphylococcus pyogenes, Staphylococcus epidermidis, Escherichia coll, Micrococcus luteus, Enterobacter aerogenes, Salmonella typhi, Pseudomonas aeruginosa, Candida albicans* and *Aspergillus niger.* Promising antioxidant and healing activity was also observed.[32]

Cassia occidentalis is a plant used by indigenous peoples and in current medicine to treat hepatotoxicity. It has analgesic, antiseptic and anti-inflammatory properties. An extract of this plant was produced and applied to rats with skin wounds, showing 95% healing and re-epithelialisation after 16 days of treatment.[90]

Almond oil *(Oleum amygdalae)* has been widely used in the medical field due to its numerous health benefits. This oil has many properties, including anti-inflammatory action, in intestinal diseases, stimulating immunity and anti-hepatotoxicity. In addition, some studies show a reduction in the incidence of colon cancer with its use. Cardiovascular benefits have also been identified with an increase in the levels of so-called "good cholesterol" (high-density lipoproteins = HDL), while reducing low-density lipoproteins (LDL). Historically, almond oil had been used in ancient China and in Greek medical schools for the treatment of xerosis, psoriasis, eczema and as a reducer of hypertrophic scars in the post-operative period, softening and rejuvenating the skin, due to its emollient and lubricating properties and great effectiveness in improving the appearance and treating dry skin.

Malva sylvestris Linn. (Malvaceae) and *Púnica granatum* Linn. (Punicaceae) are important plants in traditional Iranian medicine and have been used as a remedy against oedema and in wound healing for their antimicrobial and anti-inflammatory properties. The extract of its flowers was used to evaluate wound healing activity in rats with alloxan-induced diabetes. The effectiveness of the treatment was assessed based on the wound area. The animals treated with the extract showed a significant reduction in wound area, an organised increase in collagen, more fibroblasts and fewer inflammatory cells [80,11]

Blechnum orientale Linn (Blechnaceae) is used to treat wounds, boils, abscesses and blisters, as well as stomach pain. Its potential as a wound healer was observed after producing an aqueous extract (1% and 2%) and applying it to wound excision models in rats. The results revealed a significant reduction in wound size and a shorter average epithelialisation time and greater collagen synthesis in the group treated with the 2% aqueous extract. These results were supported by histopathological examinations of wound sections which showed greater tissue regeneration, an increase in fibroblasts and greater angiogenesis in this group, showing that the aqueous extract of *Blechnum orientale* has great potential for the treatment of skin wounds.[51,95]

The leaves of *Carapa guianensis* L. (andiroba) have been used to treat various skin problems, such as ulcers. An extract of the leaves of this plant applied topically to wounds in rats resulted in a 100 per cent reduction in the area of the lesion after 15 days of treatment. It promoted an increase in the rate of wound contraction, a higher rate of re-epithelialisation, a higher rate of granulation tissue and collagen. Herbal studies prove the anti-inflammatory and healing action of *Carapa guianensis* L.[66,100]

The healing potential of *Mallotus philippinensis* MueIL Arg fruit extract was investigated in rat wounds. As a result, greater collagen formation was observed, with few inflammatory cells in the deeper tissues. According to the authors of the study, the use of this extract is safe and effective in wound healing, and the healing effect seems to be due to the reduction in tissue damage generated.[39] .

Lonicera japonica Thunb. (Caprifoliaceae) is a plant widely used in traditional Chinese medicine to treat some infectious diseases and also used in cosmetics. Clinical findings have shown that this plant has many biological functions, including hepatoprotective, cytoprotective, antimicrobial, antioxidant, antiviral, and anti-inflammatory.[73] It has been shown to be an excellent constituent in new wound healing medicines. Its antimicrobial activity against *Staphylococcus aureus, Staphylococcus epidermidis, Escherichia coli, Candida albicans* and *Candida tropicalis* has also been proven.[26]

Other studies have evaluated the effectiveness of various medicinal plants including *Clitoria ternatea, Solanum xanthocarpum, Rubus sanctus schreb and Adhatoda vasica,* used by indigenous tribes as wound treatment remedies. All were effective in repairing and healing damaged skin, promoting skin repair, improving vascularisation and angiogenesis.[85] Good healing results were also obtained in another study using an ethanolic extract of *Solanum xanthocarpum* leaves. This plant is already used in India to treat various types of skin disease.[30] Studies have evaluated the wound healing potential of *Solanum xanthocarpum* extract in streptozotocin-induced diabetic rats. Biochemical evaluations showed a significant increase in collagen, hexosamine, hyaluronic acid, protein and DNA levels, followed by a significant decline in blood glucose, lipid peroxidation, nitric oxide and pro-inflammatory cytokine expression. According to the authors, the healing effect in diabetic rats can be attributed to the presence of chlorogenic acid in combination with other phytoconstituents.[74]

The healing activity of a methanolic extract from the leaves of *Achyranthes aspera* L. was investigated in a model of wound incision and excision in albino rats of both sexes. Using a control group treated with 1% silver sulphadiazine, both drugs were applied once a day to the wounds. Wound contraction and re-epithelialisation time were assessed in this study. They observed that all groups of rats treated with the methanolic extract of *Achyranthes aspera* L. leaves showed significantly greater wound healing activity compared to the control group of rats. Histological evaluation revealed a well-organised epidermal layer, an increase in the number of fibrocytes, a notable degree of neovascularisation and epithelialisation, which were observed after 21 days of treatment, proving the efficacy of the topical use of this plant in wound healing. According to HE et al. 2017, *Achyranthes aspera* L. has been widely used to treat various diseases, including gynaecological disorder, asthma, ophthalmia, odontalgia, haemorrhoids and abdominal tumour, and has been successfully applied in difficult wound healing processes.[37]

In another study, the healing activities of the leaves of *Pedilanthus tithymaloides* (L.) and their isolated constituents were evaluated. The leaves of this plant are widely used in Indian medicine to heal wounds, burns and mouth ulcers. Ointment made from the methanolic extract of *Pedilanthus tithymaloides* (L.) was applied to the wounds of rats and compared with a control group treated with iodine-polvidone. The effects of the formulations on wound healing were assessed by the speed of wound closure, the epithelialisation period and tensile strength. Significantly greater wound healing activity was observed in the group that used the methanolic extract of *Pedilanthus tithymaloides* (L.). Its topical application caused faster epithelialisation, significant wound contraction and an improvement in tensile strength 16 days after the start of treatment. Histological examination of tissue from groups treated with the formulation also showed complete epithelialisation with an increase in collagen, compared to the povidone-iodine control group.

The results proved the effectiveness of the traditional use of *Pedilanthus tithymaloides* (L.) for the treatment of skin wounds.[42]

Elaeagnus angustifolia (Russian olive) is one of the most widely used herbs in traditional Iranian medicine. Phytochemical studies have shown that the aqueous extract of the fruit of this plant contains flavonoid compounds, sitosterois, glycosides and terpenoids which, among other properties, accelerate wound healing. A study was carried out to prove the effect of the herb's aqueous extract on skin healing. The treated group received the plant extract, the positive control group was treated with 2% mupirocin ointment and the control group received no treatment. The results indicated that the *Elaeagnus angustifolia* extract accelerated the healing of skin wounds compared to the controls and its effect may be due to increased re-epithelialisation and collagen deposition.[63,67]

Pinus species (a type of pine tree) have been used for wound healing in Turkish folk medicine for many years. The essential oils from the cones and needles of five different Pinus species {*Pinus brutia* Ten., *Pinus halepensis* Mill., *Pinus nigra* Arn., *Pinus pinea* L. and *Pinus sylvestris* L.), were evaluated for their "in vivo" action on healing and also as an anti-inflammatory. The essential oils obtained from the cones of *Pinus pinea* L. and *Pinus halepensis* Mill showed excellent results in wound healing. *Pinus pinaster* essential oil showed excellent wound healing and anti-inflammatory effects. A-pinene was the main constituent of the essential oil obtained from the cones.[94,78,97] .

Microbial infections in wounds represent a challenge for the study of wound treatment and healing. The antimicrobial and antioxidant properties of methanolic extracts of the stem bark of *Kigelia africana* and the leaf and root of *Strophanthus hispidus* were studied to determine the wound healing properties of this plant. The influence of the extracts on the rate of wound closure was investigated using the wound excision model and histopathological investigation of the treated and untreated tissues. As a result, it was observed that methanolic extracts of the stem bark of *Kigelia africana and* the leaf and root of *Strophanthus hispidus* exhibited antimicrobial, antioxidant and wound healing effects, justifying the medicinal use of these plants for the treatment of microbial and wound infections.[3]

Sphaeranthus amaranthoides is commonly used in folk medicine to treat skin diseases. In a study to evaluate the healing activity of this plant, a methanolic extract was prepared using the whole plant and a flavonoid fraction obtained from chromatography. Wound contraction, epithelialisation period, hydroxyproline content and collagen levels were studied. As a result, the methanolic extract exhibited good wound healing activity, probably due to the presence of phenolic compounds and flavonoids. It significantly increased the rate of wound contraction and the period of epithelialisation when compared to the silver sulphadiazine control.[40]

Factors that contribute to the chronicity of wounds include trauma, poor perfusion or oxygenation and excessive inflammation. Imbalances such as in the generation of free radicals cause tissue damage and delayed healing. When tested in a study, the ethanolic extract of *Bacopa monniera* showed 50 per cent healing in chronic skin lesions in rats, probably due to the reduction of free radicals through an antioxidant effect, collagen deposition and bactericidal activity. These results prove that *Bacopa monniera* is an excellent ally in healing.[62]

The fruits of *Amorpha fruticosa* L. are used in traditional Chinese medicine to treat oedema, eczema and burns. However, little is known about the functional role of its fruits in wound healing. *In* order to prove the healing action of this plant, a study was carried out to evaluate the antimicrobial potential and wound healing activity of its fruits, both *in vitro* and *in vivo*. The results showed its great antimicrobial potential against *Bacillus subtilis, Bacillus cerculences, Staphylococcus aureus, Escherichia coli, Pseudomonas aeruginosa* and *Klebsiella aeruginosa*, and significantly increased the proliferation and migration of fibroblasts, promoting wound healing.[82]

Neurolaena lobata (Asteraceae) is a plant used in Trinidad and Tobago and the Caribbean. Its leaves contain a potent anti-parasitic agent called sesquiterpene dialdehyde, which is effective against intestinal parasites, candida and fungal infections. It is also used to control diabetes and heal wounds and infections. A study was carried out to investigate the effects of its leaf extract on wound healing in rats. The test group received the plant extract and the control group was treated with mupirocin and petroleum jelly. The result was an 87% reduction in wound area over 13 days compared to the control (78%), as well as an increase in the rate of wound contraction and a reduction in epithelialisation time in animals treated with the extract.[64,43]

Essential oils are natural substances present in plants, responsible for the aromatic odours found in them, and are obtained mainly by steam distillation. They are found in flowers, leaves, tree bark, citrus peel, roots and seeds. They have biochemical, electromagnetic and hormonal properties that are very similar and compatible with human nature. As a result, they act to harmonise and strengthen the body, both emotionally and physically.[55,70]

Complex in composition, essential oils are known to have a variety of pharmacological effects including antiviral, antimicrobial, anti-inflammatory, antioxidant, healing and cell regenerating activity.[52] Because of these properties, they are of growing interest in both industry and scientific research. They have various uses in folk medicine, as food flavourings, in perfumery, and in the pharmaceutical industry.[29,99,60 ' -70]

In recent years, there has been a considerable increase in the number of studies and scientific publications on the proven therapeutic properties of different essential oils, thus increasing their use in the manufacture of medicines and cosmetics, including dermocosmetics or cosmeceuticals (products that bring benefits to the human body, whose efficacy is proven and measured through *in vitro* and *in vivo* tests). Already well studied are clove essential oil *(Dianthus caryophyllus),* which has healing and anti-infectious properties, and tea tree oil *(Melaleuca alternifolia), which is* healing, antiseptic, fungicidal and bactericidal.[55,76,60,70]

Lavender essential oil *(Lavandula angustifolia)* is characterised by its high linalool terpenoid content. It has various properties such as: antibacterial, antifungal, moisturising, cell revitalising, healing and soothing, as well as its extremely pleasant aroma[23,15,60] . The antiseptic and medicinal qualities of aromatic plants have been recognised since ancient times, but laboratory evidence of their properties is recent (early 1900s).

According to a descriptive study carried out by Mikaili et al, 2012, traditional Iranian medicine uses various oils extracted from plants to treat different types of illnesses. The essential oil of *Carum carvi L.* (Caraway), due to its moisturising properties, is widely used with proven efficacy in the treatment of wrinkles and xerosis. The essential oil extracted from *Rosa centifolia L.,* known as Pink Cabbage and native to Iran, has, among other therapeutic properties, the ability to improve skin with xerosis, being used as a tonic and anti-inflammatory for the skin.[58]

According to the study, rose oil is obtained from the petals of different species, especially *Rosa centifolia* L. and *Rosa damascena* Mill, which have anti-inflammatory, anti-infectious and healing activities and have been used to relieve headaches, inflammatory conditions of the gastrointestinal tract and muscle pain.[58]

The properties of *Arnebia densiflora* root oil were observed in wound healing compared to Vaseline-based treatment. The group treated with the oil experienced faster healing and greater expression of growth factors and fibroblasts than the group treated with petroleum jelly.[77,5,49]

Most essential oils from plants in Brazil are obtained by steam distillation and also by pressing the pericarp of citrus fruits. Essential oils are mainly composed of mono- and sesquiterpenes and phenylpropanoids, metabolites that give them their organoleptic characteristics. Flowers, leaves, bark, rhizomes and fruit are raw materials for their production, such as the essential oils of rose, eucalyptus, cinnamon, ginger and orange, respectively. They are widely used in perfumery, cosmetics, food and as adjuvants in medicines. Brazil has a leading position in the production of essential oils, alongside India, China and Indonesia, which are considered the world's four major producers. Brazil's position is mainly due to citrus essential oils.[19]

Brazil has the largest diverse forest reserve on the planet, and many of these species used for medicinal purposes have not yet been proven to have pharmacological properties. The use of medicinal plants is not restricted to rural areas or regions without medical or pharmaceutical assistance. They are also used intensively in urban areas as an alternative or complement to allopathic medicines. The medicinal potential of a species is due to the presence of active principles capable of producing diverse pharmacological effects, such as analgesics, antiseptics, diuretics, soothing, healing, emollients, among others.

The interest in discovering new substances has led scientists from various fields to search the Brazilian flora for plant species with medicinal properties used by the population. This can be seen in the various studies evaluating the healing potential of plants capable of stimulating surgical repair. Aroeira *(Schinus terebinthifolius),* for example, a plant native to Brazil, has been used in folk medicine in the form of teas and infusions, with different properties such as: anti-inflammatory, febrifuge, analgesic and purifying agent; it has also been used as a wound healer. Many of its properties or healing effects can be attributed to the different polyphenols, which are distributed unevenly in its various organs.[88]

A study using *Schinus terebinthifolius* extract on wound healing in rats showed that the use of this extract had anti-inflammatory and angiogenic effects and improved collagen replacement. According to the authors, this plant can be used in the development of herbal medicines to treat inflammatory diseases and for wound healing.[34]

Due to the fact that many medicinal plants provide comparable results to conventional medicinal agents in the treatment of different diseases, the Brazilian government recently launched a programme known as Relação Nacional de Plantas de Interesse para o SUS (RENISUS), which lists 71 plants used in Brazilian folk medicine. The programme aims to support phytotherapy as an alternative treatment for diseases and also to encourage Brazilian researchers to validate the pharmacological properties of these plants, including their efficacy and safety. It is important to remember that in recent years the Brazilian Ministry of Health has endeavoured to encourage the inclusion of complementary care practices in the official health system. Of particular note is the implementation of the National Policy on Medicinal Plants and Herbal Medicines and the National Policy on Integrative and Complementary Practices, both in 2006, which aim to encourage access to complementary practices and medicinal plants for effective and safe health care.[81]

Sebastiania hispida, a plant species common in the Pantanal and Mato Grosso do Sul, Brazil, was the subject of a study to evaluate its effectiveness in healing wounds infected by *Staphylococcus aureus.* The authors created gels containing (0.2 and 2 per cent) *Sebastiania hispida* extract. As a result, both concentrations were effective in healing and the 0.2% gel was the most effective against the growth of S. *aureus* strains. The effectiveness in healing was possibly due to the high content of phenolic compounds, flavonoids and triterpenes.[61] .

Studies have shown that the application of phytotherapeutic agents can be highly effective in healing wounds and burns.[57] The mechanism of tissue healing is a complex biological process involving a perfect and coordinated cascade of cellular and molecular events that promote tissue reconstitution. This process arises as a tissue response to injuries induced by trauma or surgical procedures.[59]

Bixa orellana L. is a Brazilian plant native to the Amazon region, popularly known as annatto. Studies have shown that it has antibacterial, antifungal, anti-inflammatory, hyperlipidaemic, laxative, hypotensive and wound-healing properties. The aim of this study was to evaluate the action of the oily extract of *Bixa orellana L.* on the healing of skin wounds in rats. The results generated in this study show that the treatment of skin wounds with annatto seed extract is capable of accelerating the initial stages of healing. According to the authors, the use of herbal medicines is a low-cost and easily accessible alternative for treating skin wounds.[21]

Tropaeolum majus, popularly known in Brazil as chaguinha, capuchin and nasturtium, has its leaves used to treat various diseases: cardiovascular disorders, urinary tract infection, asthma, constipation, as well as its anti-inflammatory, antiseptic, antiscorbutic and antimicrobial properties. A study was carried out to evaluate the healing action of the hydroethanolic extract of the leaves of this plant on skin lesions in rats. The use of this extract improved the healing process by increasing the formation of neovessels and collagenisation.[28]

Herbal medicine containing *Aloe vera,* associated with Propolis, Copaiba oil, *Calendula (Calendula officinalis)* and Barbatim *(Stryphnodendron adstringens)* has been used on skin lesions to help the healing process and has shown excellent results. -[91,59,48]

In addition to copaiba oil, other medicinal plants that stand out for their healing properties are barbatimão and ipê roxo *(Tabebuia impetiginosa).* Barbatimão *(Stryphnodendron barbatiman* Martius) has a thick bark with an astringent effect. Its pharmacological action as a wound and ulcer healer is due to its richness in tannins. The extract of its bark contains phenolic compounds called tannins, which have antimicrobial, antioxidant and astringent properties, as they bind to proteins and polysaccharides, forming a protective layer over the lesion, stimulating re-epithelialisation.[27,25,86,59]

Calendula (Calendula officinalis L.) has been routinely used in topical applications, both in cosmetology and dermatology. Among its most widespread therapeutic attributes are the re-epithelialisation and healing of skin wounds. European folk medicine recommends its use in the treatment of eczema. The effect of the ethanolic extract of its flowers grown in Brazil was evaluated on the healing of skin wounds in rats. After 14 days of treatment, the wounds healed completely, confirming the plant's action in the process of regenerating wounds. [72,59,48,11]

pequi oil *(Caryocar brasiliense), a* fruit from the Brazilian cerrado, is rich in unsaturated fatty acids, has been used in food and in the cosmetics industry, and is indicated in popular medicine for its anti-inflammatory and healing effects and in the treatment of respiratory diseases, gastric ulcers, muscular and rheumatic pain. A study was carried out to analyse the effect of pequi oil on the healing process of skin lesions in rats. This study concluded that the use of pequi oil had a positive influence on the repair process of skin lesions in rats, as it promoted faster tissue repair.[16]

According to Castro et al. 2011, the oil extracted from the andiroba seed *(Carapa guianensis Aublet.),* which contains 60% of its mass in oil, is widely used in Brazil for its anti-inflammatory, antiseptic and anti-parasitic properties. The authors carried out a study to analyse the physico-chemical properties of this oil, as well as the acidity index, lipid distribution and presence of phyto-ingredients. They showed that andiroba oil protects the skin and helps with regeneration and healing processes. It was observed that the highest percentage of fatty acid in andiroba is oleic acid (52 per cent). This fatty acid is an additive used in soaps to give the skin lubricity and emollience. It is also widely used in cosmetic creams and emulsions due to its properties that help restore oiliness to dry skin and skin with flaking problems.[100]

Linseed oil *(Linum usitatissimum)* is used in pharmaceuticals throughout

Brazil, in the form of oil or ointment, and is indicated for use in cases of pruritic dermatoses and burns. In traditional Chinese medicine, it is used to treat wounds and as a dermal moisturiser and antioxidant, among other applications. Researchers have developed a study showing that these pharmacological properties are attributed to the presence of polyunsaturated fatty acids and monounsaturated fatty acids in its composition, which act by stimulating the production of growth factors, fibroblasts and neovascularisation. What's more, this oil has anti-inflammatory properties that guarantee optimum results in wound healing when applied topically.[38] A review of the pharmacological properties and clinical use of *Linum usitatissimum* has shown it to have antioxidant, immunomodulatory, anti-inflammatory, antimicrobial, antiprotozoal, insecticidal, analgesic, antihyperlipidaemic, antihyperglycaemic, antitumour and wound healing activity.[7]

Croton zehntneri is a Euphorbiaceae species native to north-eastern Brazil, where teas are made from its leaves and used as a healing agent. In a study aimed at proving the healing activity of this plant, excisional wounds were made on the right and left sides of the back of rats. A topical pharmaceutical formulation, developed with essential oil extracted from *Croton zehntneri* leaves (2% and 20%), was administered to the rats twice a day for 15 days. On the third day of application, it was observed that treatment with 20% of this oil reduced oedema and accelerated wound closure, with an increased number of fibroblasts and collagen fibres. The results indicate that this oil exerts significant activity in wound healing, demonstrating its relevant therapeutic potential.[22]

Aleurites moluccana L. (Willd) also a Euphorbiaceae, is a tree native to Indonesia and India, commonly used in traditional medicine to treat fever, inflammation, asthma, hepatitis, gastric ulcers, skin wounds and other diseases. The sap that flows from the stems soon after the fruit is harvested is traditionally used by Hawaiians to treat skin wounds. A study was carried out to develop a medicine based on *Aleurites moluccana* L., containing 0.5 and 1.0

per cent of the dry leaf extract of this plant, for topical use in the treatment of pain, inflammation and wound healing. As a result, both formulations proved to be effective as an analgesic, anti-inflammatory and wound-healing agent.[24] Pre-clinical studies have shown that the dry extract obtained from *Aleurites moluccana* L. leaves was effective as an analgesic, anti-inflammatory and wound healing agent, indicating that this plant is a promising herbal medicine for treating inflammatory skin diseases.[46]

Chenopodium ambrosioides (L) (Amaranthaceae) is a perennial plant popularly known as St Mary's grass, mastrux or tingling grass. It is used in folk medicine in the form of teas, poultices and infusions for inflammatory problems, wound healing, bruises, lung infections, as an anthelmintic and antifungal. Research has revealed that the plant contains terpenes, sterols and phenols. A study was carried out with the aim of proving the anti-inflammatory and healing properties of the ethanolic extract obtained from the leaves and stems of *Chenopodium ambrosioidesevn,* in animal models with skin wounds, thus validating its therapeutic use for the treatment of wounds. The results revealed that topical application of (5%) to excision wounds caused a reduction in oedema and a significant reduction in wound area, when compared to untreated controls.[96,59]

Native to the caatinga ecosystem, *Anadenanthera colubrina* VeIL Brenan, known as angico, is a plant found in the south, northeast and southeast regions of Brazil. The inner bark contains tannins with healing properties and is commonly used in folk medicine as a syrup. Its hydroalcoholic extract has antimicrobial activity "in vitro" against *Staphylococcus aureus.* A study was carried out to demonstrate the antibacterial properties of angicos and its use in folk medicine, promoting healing and tissue repair. The morphology and neoangiogenesis of skin wounds in rats treated with a 5% hydroalcoholic extract of *Anadenanthera colubrina* were assessed. As a result, the morphological analysis showed larger fibroblasts and a higher concentration of collagen fibres at seven and 14 days and the morphometric analysis showed a significant increase in the number of blood vessels over the same period in the wounds treated with the angico extract, which induced and accelerated the healing of wounds in the skin of rats.[79,78]

In a study carried out to evaluate the antibacterial and healing activity of buriti oil *(Mauritia flexuosa* L.), topical applications of a cream containing 10 per cent of this oil were made to the skin wounds of *Wistar* rats for 21 days. A significant reduction in wound area was observed on the 14th day, as well as a higher percentage of wound contraction. They also observed a significant increase in fibroblast count, collagen fibres and a complete re-epithelialisation process in the animals analysed, revealing that buriti oil is an excellent healing agent. Buriti *(Mauritia flexuosa* L.) is rich in carotenoids, polyphenols and ascorbic acid. Other studies in the literature report the healing and antioxidant potential of this oil - -[141393] ' [-12]

Euphorbia tirucalli L. (Euphorbiaceae) is known in Brazil as hazelnut. Its latex has been popularly used in traditional medicine as an anthelmintic and anti-tumour agent. Some biological properties of *this* plant have been confirmed as bactericidal and anti-herpes. These activities are probably related to the presence of phytosterols and triterpenes. In order to evaluate the effectiveness of the crude extract of this plant in healing wounds on the skin of rats, a study was carried out emphasising the macro and microscopic aspects of wound healing. The hydroalcoholic extract of *Euphorbia tirucalli* L. was applied to the wound of the study group, while the same volume of 0.9% saline solution was applied to the control group for 14 days. As a result, the group treated with the extract showed an improvement in the healing process, acute inflammation and fibrosis 14 days post-operatively.[89] *Euphorbia tirucalli* L. (Euphorbiaceae) is used in traditional medicine to treat ulcers, warts and has anti-cancer properties.[92]

Bowdichia virgilioides Kunth (Fabaceae) is a plant that grows in several South American countries, such as Venezuela, Guyana and Brazil. Various parts of this plant are used in traditional Brazilian medicine to treat illnesses. The bark is used to heal wounds, as an antiulcer and antidiabetic agent. Other parts, such as the seeds, are used in folk medicine to treat skin diseases.[33] One study evaluated the wound healing activity of *Bowdichia virgilioides* Kunth using an aqueous extract of the stem bark. Wound contraction and epithelialisation were assessed on different days using the excisional model. After nine days, the animals treated with this extract showed a significant reduction in wound area when compared to the controls that used saline solution. Wound contraction was significantly observed in the mice treated with the extract. Histological analyses showed induction of collagen deposition and an increase in fibroblast count. The expression of type I collagen was increased in the group treated with this plant, making it an excellent healing agent for skin wounds.[2]

Aroeira *(Schinus terebinthifolius* Raddi) belongs to the Anacardiaceae family and is widely used in folk medicine in Brazil, where it is found from Pernambuco to Rio Grande do Sul, and is popularly known as Brazilian pepper, aroeira or pink pepper. It is used to treat wounds and ulcers of the skin and mucous membranes, against infections of the respiratory system, digestive system and genitourinary tract. It has been the subject of several studies involving the use of extracts of its bark, leaves and fruit as a healing promoter and as an antibacterial and antifungal agent. A study aimed at evaluating the effects of an ointment containing mastic oil *(Schinus terebinthifolius)* on the healing of cutaneous wounds in rats, compared with the use of an ointment based on Vaseline and lanolin, concluded that mastic oil accelerated the wound healing process with total healing in 21 days of treatment.[34]

Studies have shown a significant effect of plasters made from *Brassica* sp leaves on the healing of skin wounds. *Brassica oleracea* is an edible vegetable whose leaves are used by the population as a healing agent for skin wounds. Despite its use in folk medicine, scientific studies of this plant are scarce. To investigate the effect of *Brassica oleracea* on the healing of skin wounds in rats, a balsam was produced using this plant. Twenty-four Wistar rats were divided into groups of animals: untreated and treated with balsam. Wounds were made on the back of all the animals. The results showed that the balsam was effective in the healing process.[84]

The leaves of *Arrabidaea chica* have aglycones, carajurin and carajurone, components of anthocyanins, with a strong pharmacological potential due to their healing properties. A study was carried out with the aim of investigating the effect of topical application of *Arrabidaea chica* leaf extract on the healing of the calcaneal tendon of Wistar rats, compared with healing using saline solution alone. As a result, they observed that the topical application of *Arrabidaea chica* extract improved the organisation of the collagen fibres, demonstrating that the extract of this plant acted on the proliferative phase of the repair of the lesion, improving the molecular organisation of the collagen fibres.[9] According to Sá and collaborators in their study to evaluate the cytotoxic, leishmanicidal and healing potential, *Arrabidaea chica* is used almost everywhere in Brazil to treat skin diseases, anaemia, jaundice and inflammatory reactions, in addition to its great leishmanicidal potential.[87,41]

Burns are serious traumas related to skin damage, causing extreme pain and even death. *Aloe vera* and vitamin E have shown beneficial effects in formulations for healing these wounds. The work by Pereira et al, 2014, aimed to develop and evaluate polymeric films containing *Aloe vera and* vitamin E to treat wounds caused by burns. Polymeric films containing different amounts of sodium alginate and polyvinyl alcohol were characterised by their mechanical properties. The polymeric films that were produced were thin, flexible, resistant and suitable for application on the damaged skin of people with burns. The results obtained showed that bioadhesive films containing vitamin E and *Aloe vera* could represent an innovative therapeutic system with excellent results in the treatment of burns.[59,11]

2.2 Bibliography

1. ABDULLA, M. A.; AHMED, K. A.; ALI, H. M. et al. Wound healing activities of Rafflesia hasseltii extract in rats. J Clin Biochem Nutr, 45: 304-308, 2009.

2. AGRA, I. K.; PIRES, L. L.; CARVALHO, P. S. et al. Evaluation of wound healing and antimicrobial properties of aqueous extract from Bowdichia virgilioides stem barks in mice. An Acad Bras de Cienc, 85(3): 945-954, 2013.

3. AGYARE, C.; DWOBENG, A. S.; AGYEPONG, N. et al. Antimicrobial, Antioxidant, and Wound Healing Properties of Kigelia africana (Lam.) Beneth. and Strophanthus hispidus DC. Adv in Pharmacol Sei, 2013(2013): 1-10, 2013.

4. AHMAD, Z. The uses and properties of almond oil. Complement Ther Clin Pract, 16(1): 10-12, 2010.

5. AKKOL E. K KOCA L.; PESIN I. et al. Exploring the wound healing activity of Arnebia densiflora (Nordm.) Ledeb. by in vivo models. J Ethnopharmacol, 124 (1): 137-141, 2009.

6. AMARAL W.; DESCHAMPS C.; MACHADO M.P. *et al.* Chamomile development, yield and quality of essential oil at different harvest ages. Rev. Bras. PL Med, 16(2):237-242, 2014.

7. ANSARI R.; Zarshenas M. M.; Dadbakhsh AH. A review on Pharmacological and clinicai aspects of Linum usitatissimum L. Curr Drug Discov Technol, 2018.

8. ARAÚJO A. L.; TEIXEIRA F. A.; LACERDA T. F. et al. Effects of topical application of pure and ozonised andiroba oil on experimentally induced wounds in horses / Effects of topical use of pure and ozonised andiroba oil on induced wounds in horses.Braz. J. Vet. Res. Anim. Sei. (Online), 54(1): 66-74, 2017.

9. ARO, A. A.; FREITAS, K. M.; FOGLIO, M. A. et al. Effect of the Arrabidaea chica extract on collagen fiber organisation during healing of partially transected tendon. Life Sei, 92(13), 799-807, 2013

10. ARRUDA J. T.; APPROBATO F. C.; MAIA M.C.S. *et al.* Effect of aqueous extract of chamomile *(Chamomilla recutita* L.) on rat pregnancy and pup development. Rev. Bras. PL Med, 15(1): 66-71,2013.

11. ATAIDE A. J.; CEFALI L. C.; CROISFELT F. M. et al. Natural actives for wound healing: A review. Phytother Res, 2018.

12. BARBOSA M. U.; SILVA M. A.; BARROS E. M. L. et al. Topical action of Buriti oil (Mauritia flexuosa L.) in myositis induced in rats. Acta Cir Bras, 32(11): 956-963, 2017.

13. BARROS E. M. L.; LIRA S. R. S.; LEMOS S. I. A. et al. Study of buriti

(Mauritia flexuosa L.) cream in the healing process / Study of buriti (Mauritia flexuosa L.) cream in the healing process. ConsSaude, 13(4), 2014.

14. BATISTA, J. S.; OLINDAI, R. G.; MEDEIROS, V. B. et al. Antibacterial and healing activity of buriti oil Mauritia flexuosa L. Ciênc Rural, 42(1): 136-141,2012.

15. BEN DJEMAA F. G.; BELLASSOUED K.; ZOUARI S. et al. Antioxidant and wound healing activity of Lavandula aspic L. ointment. J Tissue Viability, 25 (4): 193-200, 2016.

16. BEZERRA N. K. M. S.; BARROS, T. L.; COELHO, N. P. M. F. A ação do óleo de pequi (Caryocar brasiliense) no processo cicatricial de lesões cutâneas em ratos. Rev. Bras. PL Med., 17(4): 875-880, 2015.

17. BHAGAVATHULA, N.; WAGNER, R. L.; SILVA, M. et aL A combination of curcumin and ginger extract improves abrasion wound healing in corticosteroid-damaged hairless skin. Wound rep reg, 17(3): 360-366, 2009.

18. BHASKAR, A.; NITHYA, V. Evaluation of the wound-healing activity of Hibiscus rosa sinensis L (Malvaceae) in Wistar albino rats. Indian J Pharmacol, 44(6): 694-698, 2012.

19. BIZZO, R. H.; HOVELL, A. M. C.; REZENDE, C. M. Essential oils in Brazil: general aspects, development and perspectives. Quim Nova, 32(3): 588-594, 2009.

20. BODALSKA K.; HAN S.; FREIER J.; SMOLENSKI H. et al. Curcuma longa as medicinal herb in the treatment of diabetic complications. Acta Pol Pharm,74 (2): 605-610, 2017.

21. CAPELLA S. O.; TILLMANN M, T.; FÉLIX. A. O . C. et al. Healing potential of Bixa orellana L. in cutaneous wounds: study in an experimental model. Arq. Bras. Med. Vet. Zootec, 68(1): 104-112, 2016

22. CAVALCANTI, J. M.; LEAL-CARDOSO, J. H.; DINIZ, L. R. et al. The essential oil of Croton zehntneri and trans-anethole improves cutaneous wound healing. J Ethnopharnnacol., 144(2): 240-247, 2012.

23. CAVANAGH, H. M. A.; WILKINSON, J. M. Biological activities of Lavender essential oil. Phytother Res, 16(4): 301-308, 2002.

24. CESCA, T. G.; FAQUETI, L. G.; ROCHA, L. W. et al. Antinociceptive, anti-inflammatory and wound healing features in animal models treated with a semisolid herbal medicine based on aleurites moluccana l. willd. Euforbiaceae standardised leaf extract: semisolid herbal. J Ethnopharmacol, 143(1): 355-362, 2012.

25. CHAVES, D. A.; LEMES, S. R.; ARAÚJO, L. A. et al. Evaluation of the angiogenic activity of the aqueous solution of barbatimão (Stryphnodendron adstringens). Rev. Bras. Pl. Med, 18(2): 524-530, 2016.

26. CHEN, W. C., LIOU, S. S.; TZENG, T. F. et al. Wound repair and anti-inflammatory potential of Lonicera japonica in excision wound-induced rats. BMC Complement Altern Med., 12(226): 1-9, 2012.

27. COELHO, J. M.; ANTONIOLLI, A. B.; SILVA, D. N. et al. The effect of silver sulphadiazine, ipê-roxo extract and barbatimão extract on the healing of cutaneous wounds in rats. Rev Col Bras Cir, 37(1): 045- 051,2010.

28. CORRÊA, J. S.; MONTEIRO E. A.; PAVANELLI M. F. et al. Influence of the Hydroethanolic Extract of Tropaeolum majus Leaves on Tissue Restoration in Skin Lesions. Saude e pesqui. (Impr.), 9(1): 101-109, 2016.

29. DEBA, F.; XUAN, T. D.; YASUDA, M. et al. Chemical composition and antioxidant, antibacterial and antifungal activities of the essential oils from Bidens pilosa Linn. var. Radiata. Food Control, 19(4): 346-352, 2008.

30. DEWANGAN, H.; BAIS, M.; JAISWAL, V. et al. Potential wound healing activity of the ethanolic extract of Solanum Xanthocarpum schrad and wendl leaves. Pak J Pharm Sei, 25(1): 189-194, 2012.

31. DRAGOS D.; GILCA M.; GAMAN L. et al. Phytomedicine in joint disorders. Nutrients, 9 (1): 2-18, 2017.

32. DWIVEDI D.; DWIVEDI M.; MALVIYA S. et al. Evaluation of wound healing, anti-microbial and antioxidant potential of Pongamia pinnata in wistar rats. J Tradit Complement Med, 7(1): 79-85, 2016.

33. ENDO Y.; KASAHARA T.; HARADA K. et al. Sucupiranins A-L, Furanocassane Diterpenoids from the Seeds of Bowdichia virgilioides. J. Nat. Prod, 80, 3120-3127, 2017.

34. ESTEVÃO, L. R. M.; SIMÕES R. S.; CASSINI-VIEIRA P. et al. Schinus terebinthifolius Raddi (Aroeira) leaves oil attenuates inflammatory responses in cutaneous wound healing in mice. Acta Cir. Bras, 32(9): 726-735, 2017.

35. FAN B.; WANG T.; BIAN L. et al. Topical Application of Tat-Rac1 Promotes Cutaneous Wound Healing in Normal and Diabetic Mice. Int J Biol Sei, 14(10):1163-1174, 2018.

36. FEDERICI, A.; FEDERICI, G.; MILANI, M. An urea and carnosine based cream (Ureadin Rx Db ISDIN) shows greater efficacy in the treatment of severe xerosis of the feet in type 2 diabetic patients in comparison with glycerol-based emollient cream. BMC Dermatol, 12(1): 16, 2012.

37. FIKRU, A.; MAKONNEN, E.; EGUALE, T. et al. Evaluation of in vivo wound healing activity of methanol extract of Achyranthes aspera L. J Ethnopharmacol, 143(2): 469-474, 2012.

38. FRANCO, E. S.; AQUINO, C. M. F.; MEDEIROS, P. L. et al. Effect of a Semisolid Formulation of Linum usitatissimum L. (Linseed) Oil on the Repair of Skin Wounds. Evid Based Complement Alternat Med, 2012: 17, 2012.

39. GANGWAR M.; GAUTAM MK.; GHILDIYAL S. et al. Mallotus philippinensis MuelL Arg fruit glandular hairs extract promotes wound healing on different wound model in rats. BMC Complement Altern Med, 15: 123, 2015.

40. GEETHALAKSHMI, R.; SAKRAVARTHI, C.; KRITIKA, T. et al. Evaluation of Antioxidant and Wound Healing Potentials of Sphaeranthus amaranthoides Burm.f. Biomed Res, 2013(2013): 1-7, 2013.

41. GEMELLI T. F.; PRADO I. S.; SANTOS F. S. et al. Evaluation of Safety of Arrabidaea chica Verlot(Bignoniaceae), a Plant with Healing Properties. J Toxicol Environ Health A, 2015; 78 (18): 1170-80

42. GHOSH, S.; SAMANTA, A.; MANDAL, N. B. et al. Evaluation of the wound healing activity of methanol extract of Pedilanthus tithymaloides (L.) Poit leaf and its isolated active constituents in topical formulation. J Ethnopharmacol, 142(3): 714-22, 2012.

43. GIOVANNINI P.; HOWES M. R .; EDWARDS S. E. Medicinal plants used in the traditional management of diabetes and its sequelae in Central America: a review. J Ethnopharmacol, 7: 1217-1220, 2016.

44. GUPTA, A.; UPADHYAY, N. K.; SAWHNEY, R. C. et al. Poly-herbal formulation accelerates normal and impaired diabetic wound healing. Wound Repair Regen, 16(6): 784-790, 2008.

45. HAYOUNI, E. A.; MILED, K.; BOUBAKER, S. et al. Hydroalcoholic extract based-ointment from Púnica granatum L. peeis with enhanced in vivo healing potential on dermal wounds. Phytomedicine, 18(11): 976- 984, 2011.

46. HOEPERS S.; MARTINS G. H.; SOUZA T. et al. Topical anti- inflammatory activity of semisolid containing standardised Aleurites moluccana L. WILLD (EUPHORBIACEAE) leaves extract. J Ethnopharmacol, 173: 251-255, 2015.

47. HOSSEINKHANI A.; FALAHATZADEH M.; RAOOFI E. et al. An Evidence-Based Review on Wound Healing Herbal Remedies From Reports of Traditional Persian Medicine. J Evid Based Complementary Altern Med, 2017.

48. JARIC S.; KOSTIC O.; MATARUGA Z. et al. Traditional wound-healing plants used in the Balkan region (Southeast Europe). J Ethnopharmacol, 211:311-328, 2018.

49. KOSGER H. H.; OZTURK M.; SOKMEN A. et al. Wound healing effects of arnebia densiflora root extracts on rat palatal mucosa. Eur J Dent, 3 (2): 96-99, 2009.

50. KUMAR, B.; VIJAYAKUMAR, M.; GOVINDARAJAN, R. et al. Ethnopharmacological approaches to wound healing-Exploring medicinal plants of India. J Ethnopharmacol, 114(2): 103-113, 2007.

51. LAI, H. Y.; LIM, Y. Y.; KIM, K. H. et al. Potential dermal wound healing agent in Blechnum orientale Linn. BMC Complement Altern Med., 11(62): 1-5, 2011.

52. LEE, S. B.; CHA, K. H.; KIM, S. N. et al. The antimicrobial activity of essential oil from Dracocephalum foetidum against pathogenic microorganisms. J Microbiol, 45(1): 53-57, 2007.

53. MAHBOUBI M.; TAGHIZADEH M KHAMECHIAN T. et al. The Wound Healing Effects of Herbal Cream Containing Oliveria Decumbens and PelargoniumGraveolens Essential Oils in Diabetic Foot Ulcer Model. World. J Plast Surg, 7(1): 45-50, 2018.

54. MALHEIROS F. B. M.; GARCIA A. C.; SOUZA L. M. A. et al. Healing effect of the fluid extract of Chamomilla recutita (L.) Rauschert in magisterial semi-solid formulas applied to skin lesions in rats. ConScientiae Saúde, 2011;10(3):425-432.

55. MALUFE, S.; AJAUSKAS, M. C. The use of essential oils in podiatry and aromatherapy. RevistaPodologia, (14): 21-26, 2007.

56. MARTINO O.; TITO A.; DE LUCIA A. et al. Hibiscus syriacus Extract from an Established Cell Culture Stimulates Skin Wound Healing. Biomed Res Int, 2017.

57. MENDONÇA, F. A. S.; PASSARINI, JÚNIOR, J. R.; ESQUISATTO, M. A. et al. Effects of the application of Aloe vera (L.) and microcurrent on the healing of wounds surgically induced in Wistar rats. Acta Cir Bras, 24(2): 150-155, 2009.

58. MOHEBITABAR S.; SHIRAZI2 M.; BIOOS1 S. et al. Therapeutic efficacy of rose oil: A comprehensive review of clinical evidence. Avicenna J Phytomed, 7(3): 206-213, 2017.

59. MORESKI D. B.; BUENO F. G.; LEITE-MELLO E. V. S. Healing action of medicinal plants: a review study. Arq. Ciênc. Saúde UNIPAR, 22(1): 63-69, 2018.

60. MORI H. M.; KAWANAMI H.; KAWAHATA H. et al. Wound healing potential of lavender oil by acceleration of granulation and wound contractionthrough induction of TGF-p in a rat model. BMC Complement Altern Med, 16:144, 2016.

61. MULLER J. A. L; MATIAS R.; GUILHERMINO J. F. et al. The effect of Sebastiania hispida gel on wound model infected by methicillin resistantStaphylococcus aureus. Biomed Pharmacother, 105: 1311- 1317, 2018.

62. MURTHY, S.; GAUTAM, M. K.; GOEL, S. et al. Evaluation of In Vivo Wound Healing Activity of Bacopa monniera on Different Wound Model in Rats. Biomed Res, 2013(2013): 1-9, 2013.

63. NATANZI, M. M.; PASALAR, P.; KAMALINEJAD, M. et al. Effect of

aqueous extract of Elaeagnus angustifolia fruit on experimental cutaneous wound healing in rats. Acta Med Ira, 50(9): 589-596, 2012.

64. NAYAK, B. S. et al. Neurolaena lobata L. promotes wound healing in Sprague Dawley rats. Int J Appl Basic Med Res, 4(2): 106-110, 2014.

65. NAYAK, B. S.; RAJU, S. S.; RAO, A. V. Wound healing activity of Matricaria recutita L. extract. J Wound Care, 16(7): 298-302, 2007.

66. NAYAK, B.S. et al. Experimental Evaluation of Ethanolic Extract of Carapa guianensis L. Leaf for Its Wound Healing Activity Using Three Wound Models. Evid Based Complement Alternat Med, 8(1): 1-6, 2011.

67. NIKNAM F.; AZADI A.; BARZEGAR A. et al. Phytochemistry and Phytotherapeutic Aspects of Elaeagnus angustifolia L. Curr Drug Discov Technol, 13(4): 199-210, 2016.

68. OLIVEIRA, S. H. S.; SOARES, M. G. O.; PRADINES, S. M. S. et al. Debridement gel and associated occlusive dressing in the treatment of ulcers. MBM Farmacêutica, 2010.
Available at :
http://www.mbmfarmaceutica.com.br/ index.ph. Accessed on: 8 January 2013.

69. ORYAN A.; MOHAMMADALIPOUR A.; MOSHIRI A. *et al.* Topical Application of Aloe vera Accelerated Wound Healing, Modelling, and Remodeling: An Experimental Study. Ann Plast Surg± 77(1): 37-46, 2016.

70. PANDINI J. A.; PINTO F. G. S.; SCUR M. C. et al. Chemical composition, antimicrobial and antioxidant potential of the essential oil of Guareakunthiana A. Juss. Braz J Biol, 78(1): 53-60, 2018.

71. PAPANAS, N.; MALTEZOS, E. Polyherbal formulation as a therapeutic option to improve wound healing in the diabetic foot. Indian J Med Res, 134: 146-147, 2011.

72. PARENTE, L. M. L.; SILVA, M. S. B.; BRITO, L. A. B. et al. Healing effect and antibacterial activity of Calendula officinalis L. cultivated in Brazil. Rev Bras Pl Med, 11(4): 383-391, 2009.

73. PARK C.; LEE W. S.; HAN M. H. et al. Lonicera japonica Thunb. Induces caspase-dependent apoptosis through death receptors and suppression of AKT in U937 human leukemic cells. Phytother Res, 32(3):504-513, 2017.

74. PARMAR K. M.; SHENDE P. R.; KATARE N. et al. Wound healing potential of Solanum xanthocarpum in streptozotocin-induced diabetic rats. J Pharm Pharmacol, 2018.

75. PATON, J. S.; STENHOUSE, E. A.; BRUCE, G. et al. A comparison of customized and prefabricated insoles to reduce risk factors for neuropathic diabetic foot ulceration: a participant-blinded randomised controlled trial. J

Foot Ankle Res, 5: 1-11,2012.

76. PAZYAR, N.; YAGHOOBI, R.; BAGHERANI, N. et al. A Review of applications of tea tree oil in dermatology. Int J Dermatol, 52(7): 784-790, 2013.

77. PEI, X. W.; WANG, K. Z.; DANG, X. Q. et al. Arnebia root oil promotes wound healing and expression of basic fibroblast growth factor on the wound surface in rabbits. J Integr Med, 4(1): 52-55, 2006.

78. PÉREZ-RECALDE M.; RUIZ ARIAS I. E.; HERMIDA É. B. Could essential oils enhance biopolymers performance for wound healing? A systematic review. Phytomedicine, 38:57-65, 2018.

79. PESSOA, W. S.; ESTEVÃO, L. R.; SIMÕES, R. S. et al. Effects of angico extract (Anadenanthera colubrina var. cebil) in cutaneous wound healing in rats. Acta Cir Bras, 27(10): 655-670, 2012.

80. PIRBALOUTI, A. G.; AZIZI, S.; KOOHPAYEH, A. et al. Wound healing activity of Malva sylvestris and Púnica granatum in alloxan-induced diabetic rats. Acta Pol Pharm, 67(5): 511-516, 2010.

81. PIRIZ, M. A.; LIMA, C.A.B.; JARDIM, V. M. R. et al. Medicinal plants in the wound healing process: a literature review. Rev Bras Pl Med, 16(3): 628-636, 2014.

82. QU, X.; DIAO, Y.; ZHANG, Z. et al. Evaluation of anti-bacterial and wound healing activity of the fruits of Amorpha fruticosa L. Afr J Tradit Complement Altern Med, 10(3): 458-468, 2013.

83. RAJKUMAR S. R. J.; GNANAVEL G.; NADAR M. S. A. M. et al. wound healing activity of Morinda tinctoria Roxb aqueous leaf extract. Biotech, 8:343, 2018.

84. REBOLLA, A.; ARISAWA, E. A. S.; BARJA, P. R. et al. Effect of Brassica oleracea in rats skin wound healing. Acta Cir Bras, 28(9): 664-669, 2013.

85. REDDY, G. A. K.; PRIYANKA, B.; SARANYA, C. S. et al. Wound healing pontential of Indian medicinal plants. IJPRR, 2(2): 75-87, 2012.

86. RODRIGUES D. F.; MENDES F. F.; CARVALHO W. L. et al. Arq. Bras. Med. Vet. Zootec, 69(5): 1243-1250, 2017.

87. SÁ C. J.; SOUZA F. A.; OLIVEIRA R. M. et al. Leishmanicidal, cytotoxicity and wound healing potential of Arrabidaea chica Verlot. BMC Complement Altern Med, 16:1,2016.

88. SANTOS, O. J.; TORRES, O. J. M. The evolution of phytotherapy in surgical healing. Arq Bras Cir Dig, 25(3): 139, 2012.

89. SAUAIA FILHO, E.N.; SANTOS, O. J.; BARROS FILHO, A. K. D. et al. Evaluation of the use of raw extract of Euphorbia tirucalli L. in the healing process of skin wounds in mice. Acta Cir Bras, 28(10): 716-720, 2013.

90. SHEEBA, M.; EMMANUEL, S.; REVATHI, K. et al. Wound healing activity

of Cassia occidentalis L. in albino wistar rats. IJIB, 8(1): 1-6, 2009.

91. SHIMIZU, B. J.; EURIDES, D.; BELETTI, M. E. et al. Barbatimão extract at 5% in hydroxyethylcellulose gel applied to cutaneous wounds, experimentally produced in mice. Vet Not, 15(1): 21-27, 2009.a

92. SILVA V.A. O.; ROSA M. N.; MIRANDA G. V. et al. Euphol, a tetracyclic triterpene,from Euphorbia tirucalli induces autophagy and sensitizestemozolomide cytotoxicity on glioblastoma cells. Invest New Drugs, 2018

93. SPERANZA P.;, FALCÃO A. O.; MACEDO J. A. et al. Amazonian Buriti oil: Chemical characterisation and antioxidant potential. CSIC, 6(2): 2016

94. SÚNTAR, L; TUMEN, I.; USTUN, O. et al. Appraisal on the wound healing and anti-inflammatory activities of the essential oils obtained from the cones and needles of Pinus species by in vivo and in vitro experimental models. J Ethnopharmacol, 139(2): 533-540, 2012.

95. TAN S. T.; ONG H. C.; CHAI T. T. et al. Identification of Potential Anticancer Protein Targets in Cytotoxicity Mediated by TropicalMedicinal Fern Extracts. Pharmacogn Mag, (54): 227-230, 2018.

96. TRIVELLATOGRASSI, L.; MALHEIROS, A.; SILVA, C. M. et al. From popular use to pharmacological validation: a study of the anti-inflammatory, anti-nociceptive and healing effects of Chenopodium ambrosioides extract. J Ethnopharmacol, 145(1): 127-138, 2013.

97. TÚMEN I.; AKKOL E. K.; TAÇTAN H. et al. Research on the antioxidant, wound healing, and anti-inflammatory activities and the phytochemical composition of maritime pine (Pinus pinaster Ait). J Ethnopharmacol, 211:235-246, 2018.

98. VISWANATHAN, V.; KESAVAN, R.; KAVITHA, K. V. et al. A pilot study on the effects of a polyherbal formulation cream on diabetic foot ulcers. Indian J Med Res, 134: 168-173, 2011.

99. WANG, J.; LIU, H.; ZHAO, J. et al. Antimicrobial and Antioxidant Activities of the Root Bark Essential Oil of Periploca sepium and Its Main Component 2-Hydroxy-4-methoxybenzaldehyde. Molecules, 15: 5807-5817, 2010.

100.WANZELER A. M. V.; JÚNIOR S. M. A.; GOMES J. T. et al. Therapeutic effect of andiroba oil (Carapa guianensis Aubl.) against oral mucositis: an experimental study in golden Syrian hamsters. Clin Oral Investig, 22(5):2069-2079, 2018.

101.WICAKSONO A.; MURSIDAWATI S.; SUKAMTO L. A et al. Rafflesia spp.: propagation and conservation. Planta, 244(2): 289-296, 2016.

2.3 Index of cited plants

saffron34
Achyranthes aspera37 , 38
Adhatoda vasica37
Aleurites moluccana48
Aloe barbadensis32
Aloe vera31 , 32, 33, 46, 53
indianberry33
Amorpha fruticosa40
Anadenanthera colubrina49
andiroba36 , 47
angico49
Arnebia densiflora43
arnica32
Arnica Montana. 32
mastic13 , 32, 44, 51
Arrabidaea chica52
hazelnut50
Azadirachta indica32
olive oil32
russian olive39
babassu32
babosa32
Bacopa monniera40
barbatim13 , 32, 46
Bixa orellana45
Blechnum orientale36
Bowdichia virgilioides51
Brassica napus19
Brassica oleracea52
buriti50
Caesalpinia ferrea32
marigold32 , 46
Calendula officinalis32 , 46
chamomile34
cinnamon43
canola19
capuchin46
Carapa guianensis36 , 47
Carica papaya32
Carum carvi42
Caryocar brasiliense47
Cassia occidentalis35
chew49
mastruz32
Matricaria chamomilla34
Matricaria recutita34
Matricaria suaveolens34
Mauritia flexuosa50
melaleuca42
Melaleuca alternifolia42
Morinda citrifolia33
Morinda tinctoria33
Musa paradisiaca31

Catharanthus roseu32
Celosia argentea32
Centella asiatica32
chaguinha46
Chamomilla chamomile34
Chenopodium ambrosioides 32, 49
Cinnamomum zeylanicum32
Clitoria ternatea37
Cocos nucifera31
copaiba13 , 46
Copaifera langsdorffii13
Coronopu didymus32
carnation42
Croton zehntneri48
Curcuma longa31 , 32, 33, 34
Dianthus caryophyllus42
Elaeagnus angustifolia39
St Mary's grass32 , 49
anthill grass49
eucalyptus43
Euphorbia tirucalli50
ginger34 , 43
sunflower13 , 32
Glycyrrhiza glabra31
Helianthus annus32
Helianthus annuus13
Hibiscus rosa sinensis33
Hibiscus syriacus34
Hippophae rhamnoides32 , 33
ipê roxo32 , 46
jasmine32
Jatropha curcas32
jucá32
Kigelia africana39
orange43
lavender42
Lavandula angustifolia42
linseed47
Linum usitatissimum47
Lonicera japonica36
Mallotus philippinensis36
Malva sylvestris35
Pterocarpus santalinus32
Punica granatum35
Rafflesia hasseltii34
Pink cabbage42
rose43
Rosa centifolia42
Rosa damascena43
Rubus sanctus37
willow30
Salix alba30
Salix alba Caerulea30

nasturtium46
Nelumbo nucifera32
Neurolaena lobata41
Ocimum sanctum32
Olea europaea32
almond oil35
Oleum amygdalae35
Oliveria decombens33
Orbignya phalerata32
oregano32
Origanum vulgare32
Pandanus odaratissimus31
Pedilanthus tithymaloides38
Pelargonium graveolens33
pequi47
Phyllanthus emblica32
Brazilian chilli pepper51
pink peppercorns51
pine39
Pinus brutia39
Pinus halepensis39
Pinus nigra39
Pinus pinaster39
Pinus pinea39
Pinus sylvestris39
Plumbago zeylanica32
Pongamia Pinnata34

Salix babylonica30
Salix matsudana30
Salix sepulcralis Chrysocoma 30
Salix Tristis30
sage32
Salvia officinalis32
Schinus terebinthifolius 32, 44, 51
Schinusmolle13
Sebastiania hispida45
Solanum xanthocarpum37
Sphaeranthus amaranthoides 40
Strophanthus hispidus39
Stryphnodendron adstringens32, 46
Stryphnodendron barbatiman13, 46
Tabebuia avellanedae32
Tabebuia impetiginosa46
Tabernaemontana catharinensis 32
tea tree42
Terminalia arjuna32
Terminalia chebula32
wheat32
Triticum vulgare32
Tropaeolum majus46
annatto45
vinca rosea32
Zingiber officinalis34

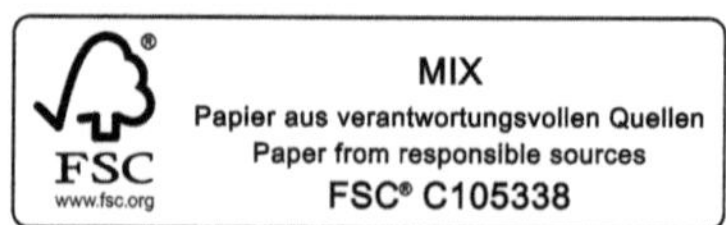

Printed by Books on Demand GmbH, Norderstedt / Germany